Phototherapy and Photochemotherapy of Skin Disease

BASIC AND CLINICAL DERMATOLOGY

Series Editors
ALAN R. SHALITA, M.D.
Distinguished Teaching Professor and Chairman
Department of Dermatology
SUNY Downstate Medical Center
Brooklyn, New York
DAVID A. NORRIS, M.D.
Director of Research
Professor of Dermatology
The University of Colorado
Health Sciences Center
Denver, Colorado

1. Cutaneous Investigation in Health and Disease: Noninvasive Methods and Instrumentation, *edited by Jean-Luc Lévêque*
2. Irritant Contact Dermatitis, *edited by Edward M. Jackson and Ronald Goldner*
3. Fundamentals of Dermatology: A Study Guide, *Franklin S. Glickman and Alan R. Shalita*
4. Aging Skin: Properties and Functional Changes, *edited by Jean-Luc Lévêque and Pierre G. Agache*
5. Retinoids: Progress in Research and Clinical Applications, *edited by Maria A. Livrea and Lester Packer*
6. Clinical Photomedicine, *edited by Henry W. Lim and Nicholas A. Soter*
7. Cutaneous Antifungal Agents: Selected Compounds in Clinical Practice and Development, *edited by John W. Rippon and Robert A. Fromtling*
8. Oxidative Stress in Dermatology, *edited by Jürgen Fuchs and Lester Packer*
9. Connective Tissue Diseases of the Skin, *edited by Charles M. Lapière and Thomas Krieg*
10. Epidermal Growth Factors and Cytokines, *edited by Thomas A. Luger and Thomas Schwarz*
11. Skin Changes and Diseases in Pregnancy, *edited by Marwali Harahap and Robert C. Wallach*
12. Fungal Disease: Biology, Immunology, and Diagnosis, *edited by Paul H. Jacobs and Lexie Nall*
13. Immunomodulatory and Cytotoxic Agents in Dermatology, *edited by Charles J. McDonald*
14. Cutaneous Infection and Therapy, *edited by Raza Aly, Karl R. Beutner, and Howard I. Maibach*

Phototherapy and Photochemotherapy of Skin Disease

THIRD EDITION

Warwick L. Morison
The Johns Hopkins School of Medicine
Baltimore, Maryland, U.S.A.

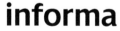

informa
healthcare

New York   London

First published in 2005 by Taylor & Francis Group.

This edition published in 2011 by Informa Healthcare, Telephone House, 69-77 Paul Street, London EC2A 4LQ, UK.

Simultaneously published in the USA by Informa Healthcare, 52 Vanderbilt Avenue, 7th Floor, New York, NY 10017, USA.

Informa Healthcare is a trading division of Informa UK Ltd. Registered Office: 37–41 Mortimer Street, London W1T 3JH, UK. Registered in England and Wales number 1072954.

A CIP record for this book is available from the British Library.

Library of Congress Cataloging-in-Publication Data available on application

ISBN-13: 978-1-5744-4880-1

Orders may be sent to: Informa Healthcare, Sheepen Place, Colchester, Essex CO3 3LP, UK
Telephone: +44 (0)20 7017 5540
Email: CSDhealthcarebooks@informa.com
Website: http://informahealthcarebooks.com/

For corporate sales please contact: CorporateBooksIHC@informa.com
For foreign rights please contact: RightsIHC@informa.com
For reprint permissions please contact: PermissionsIHC@informa.com

To my patients,
who are always teaching me something new
and to
John A. Parrish, M.D.
and the late Thomas B. Fitzpatrick, M.D., Ph.D.
pioneers in
the field of phototherapy and
photochemotherapy of skin disease

Series Introduction

During the past 25 years, there has been a vast explosion in new information relating to the art and science of dermatology as well as fundamental cutaneous biology. Furthermore, this information is no longer of interest only to the small but growing specialty of dermatology. Scientists from a wide variety of disciplines have come to recognize both the importance of skin in fundamental biological processes and the broad implications of understanding the pathogenesis of skin diseases. As a result, there is now a multidisciplinary and worldwide interest in the progress of dermatology.

With these factors in mind, we have undertaken this series of books specifically oriented to dermatology. The scope of the series is purposely broad, with books ranging from pure basic science to practical, applied clinical dermatology. Thus, while there is something for everyone, all volumes in the series will ultimately prove to be valuable additions to the dermatologist's library.

The latest addition to the series, volume 34, authored by Dr. Warwick Morison, is both timely and pertinent. The author is a well-known authority in the field of phototherapy and photochemotherapy. We trust that this volume will be of broad interest to scientists and clinicians alike.

Alan R. Shalita
SUNY Downstate Medical Center
Brooklyn, New York

Preface

The third edition of this book has the same overall aim as the first two editions: to be a practical handbook for physicians and other medical personnel interested in using UV therapy. It is not meant to be an academic tome but instead is based on 30 years of experience practicing phototherapy blended with an appraisal of the many hundreds of published studies on the subject.

There have been dramatic changes in the use of light to treat skin disease in the past decade and these changes are reflected in this reorganized and updated edition. The most important innovation has been narrowband (311 nm) UV phototherapy. First introduced more than 20 years ago, it became available in North America only 7 years ago and is an effective alternative to PUVA therapy for psoriasis and other diseases in many patients. Protocols for this treatment, its therapeutic spectrum, advantages, and limitations are described in detail. The introduction of targeted therapy using high-output sources such as the excimer laser for treatment of localized psoriasis is an outgrowth of this new modality using a similar wavelength (308 nm) and providing opportunities to treat disease of the scalp and other areas previously off limits to phototherapy. Coupled with these changes has been a declining use of PUVA therapy due particularly to concern about adverse effects such as melanoma, photoaging, and squamous cell carcinoma. This treatment may be in decline but it is not dead since it retains many advantages for the therapist and patients; a balanced evaluation of present and safe use of PUVA therapy is presented. There are some emerging new modalities such as UVA-1 phototherapy and use of light to treat acne and the most recent information on these treatments is evaluated.

More than 60% of the book has been revised and several new chapters have been added. Phototherapy for psoriasis is often used as a combination treatment rather than a monotherapy and this is reflected in the addition of a separate chapter for this subject. Introduction of the so-called biologic treatments for psoriasis make combination therapy even more important since they are likely to influence use of phototherapy and vice versa. Similarly, phototherapy is not just a treatment for psoriasis and this is emphasized because more than 40% of patients receiving this treatment may not have psoriasis as it has become the standard of care for more than 30 other diseases. A separate chapter on treatment of children has been included since there are many aspects to their treatment that are different from adult therapy.

This edition has been extensively reorganized with two aims. First, greater integration of basic principles into the "practical" chapters to allow easier understanding of protocols, problems, and their solutions. Second, many new tables have been added to highlight important information and concepts. Finally, new attention has been focused on the economics of the delivery of phototherapy since without attention to the bottom line this treatment can easily go the way of the Dodo bird.

Warwick L. Morison

Acknowledgment

I am greatly indebted to the staff in my office who have "carried the load" while I have been distracted by writing this book and who, through their questioning attitude and interest, ensure that there is always something new to learn. Ms. Vicki Dippold was an enormous help in typing and organizing the book.

Contents

Basic Principles of Photobiology

An understanding of the principles underlying phototherapy and photochemotherapy is essential for the effective use of these treatments. Many patients can be treated using the schedules that are outlined in this book without reference to the section on basic principles. With that approach, however, the treatment will not be delivered with maximum benefit, and the reasons why some patients do not respond will tend to remain a mystery. It is equally important to emphasize that every therapist does not have to become a photobiologist, physicist, and engineer just to be able to treat patients. Thus, the section on basic principles has been restricted to those concepts thought to be important for the practicing therapist. If further details are required, they are readily available in more complete photobiology textbooks.

1

Electromagnetic Radiation

INTRODUCTION

Electromagnetic radiation is a form of energy derived from the sun or produced artificially. Radiation can be characterized in two ways and although this is confusing at first glance, it does have specific usefulness. The wave description views radiation as a continuous wave propagated through space having a frequency in time and length. The wavelength is the distance between two corresponding points on successive waves. The wave theory of radiation is most useful for understanding optics such as how radiation is reflected or refracted. The particle description views radiation as discrete packages of energy called photons. This theory is most suitable for explaining photobiologic phenomena such as absorption of radiation by molecules.

WAVEBANDS

Electromagnetic radiation is divided into various regions with the broad divisions being based on differing physical, chemical, and biologic effects (Fig. 1). Wavelengths longer than 100 nm are termed "nonionizing" radiation because the energy of these photons is insufficient to cause ionization of atoms in solution.

The UV and visible portions of the electromagnetic spectrum are of most interest in photomedicine since the absorption of this energy by molecules and atoms is responsible for the various biologic responses observed.

3

ELECTROMAGNETIC SPECTRUM
WITH EXPANDED SCALE OF ULTRAVIOLET LIGHT

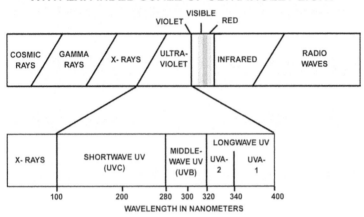

Figure 1 Electromagnetic radiation.

These wavelengths are most conveniently measured in nanometers ($1 \, nm = 10^{-9} \, m$).

Vacuum UV (100–200 nm)

These are the shortest wavelengths of UV radiation and are called vacuum UV because these photons are absorbed by air and therefore can be used experimentally only in vacuum. These wavelengths are of no interest in medical photobiology.

UVC Radiation (200–290 nm)

Radiation in the UVC waveband is not found in sunlight at the surface of the earth, as it is filtered out by ozone and water vapor in the atmosphere. Other terms for the waveband are "germicidal radiation," since it is used to kill microorganisms, and "short-wave UV," because it contains the shortest wavelengths of UV radiation. UVC radiation is often used synonymously with 254 nm radiation, because it is the main wavelength emitted by low-pressure mercury lamps. These lamps are not used in phototherapy. However, physicians may encounter germicidal lamps in operating rooms and dialysis units, where they are used for sterilization purposes, and in biology laboratories, where they are frequently used as a source of UV radiation for in vitro experiments. Biologists often refer to germicidal lamps as simply a UV lamp. Thus, when *Science* magazine reports on activation of black-eyed Susan virus by UV radiation, careful reading of the fine print will reveal that this momentous effect was induced by UVC radiation. Whether such results have any relevance to humans in their UVC-free environment is questionable at best.

UVB Radiation (290–320 nm)

UVB is the most biologically active waveband of UV radiation in sunlight and is mainly responsible for the erythemal reaction following exposure to the sun. It is also termed "middle-wave UV" or "sunburn UV radiation." The emission spectrum of a sunlamp fluorescent bulb is often considered to be limited to UVB radiation but this is untrue. Forty percent of the energy emitted by a sunlamp bulb is UVA radiation and, in addition, it also emits a small but biologically significant amount of UVC radiation.

UVA Radiation (320–400 nm)

The longest wavelengths of UV radiation are less biologically active than UVB radiation, but the UVA waveband is partially responsible for sun-induced erythema and pigmentation. Other terms for this waveband are "long-wave UV radiation," for obvious reasons; "near-UV radiation," as it is adjacent to visible light; and "black light," because it cannot be seen. Recently, the UVA waveband has been subdivided into UVA-1 (340–400 nm) and UVA-2 (320–340 nm). The reason for this division is that the two wavebands induce different photochemical reactions in DNA and other molecules. UVA-1 induces mainly oxygen-dependent photochemistry while UVA-2 induces UVB-type photochemistry with direct absorption by DNA molecules.

Visible Light

A point on terminology: "light" refers only to visible radiation, or radiation that the eye can see, and "radiation" is the correct term for other wavelengths, e.g., UV radiation and infrared radiation. The visible spectrum is usually considered to be 400–760 nm; although the retina is sensitive to wavelengths down to 350 nm, these UV wavelengths are ordinarily absorbed by the ocular media. Most observers recognize six regions of color or hues within the visible spectrum, and their ranges are given in Table 1.

ENERGY OF PHOTONS

The energy of photons is inversely proportional to the wavelength (Fig. 2) and therefore the longer the wavelength, the less energy possessed by each photon. The energy of photons is a major determinant of their biologic activity, so the shorter wavelengths in the solar spectrum produce the most biologic response. Wavelengths around 300 nm in sunlight are responsible for most of the erythema and tanning seen in human skin and due to the

Table 1 Wavebands of Colors

Color name	Range (nm)
Violet	400–440
Blue	440–500
Green	500–550
Yellow	550–590
Orange	590–650
Red	650–760

rapid fall in photon energy, wavelengths longer than 320 nm make only a small contribution to these responses.

In the presence of a photosensitizer the situation can be quite different. For example, 340 nm photons by themselves are not very biologically active but in the presence of a photosensitizer such as psoralen, the same photons are biologically very active. Similarly, photons of visible light alone can only rattle molecules but in the presence of a photosensitizing dye they can produce significant biologic effects.

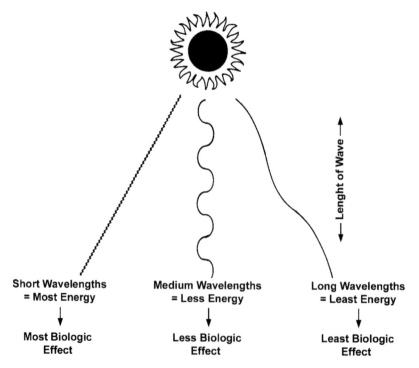

Figure 2 Energy of photons is inversely proportional to wavelength.

UNITS OF MEASUREMENT

Many different industries and occupations are interested in light and other types of nonionizing radiation and this has led to several systems of measurement. The result: much confusion. Some physicians using phototherapy still measure dosimetry in minutes and seconds, a primitive approach that assumes a constant output from a radiation source and this is seldom true. Photometric units are used to describe visible light sources and are the province of the lighting industry. In photomedicine, the system of measurement is based on radiometric units since it involves ultraviolet and infrared radiation as well as visible light. The units of measurement of interest in phototherapy are:

- Radiant energy is the amount of electromagnetic radiation and is expressed in joules (J), $1 \text{ J} = 10^3 \text{ mJ}$.
- Radiant power is the rate at which radiant energy is delivered, or energy per unit time, and is expressed in watts (W), $1 \text{ W} = 1 \text{ J}/\text{sec}$, $1 \text{ W} = 10^3 \text{ mW}$. Another term used for radiant power is radiant flux.
- Irradiance is radiant power per unit area at a given surface and is expressed as watts per square centimeter. In phototherapy practice, the irradiance of a radiation source is measured with a radiometer and the reading is given in watts per square centimeter or milliwatts per square centimeter. The reading will obviously be influenced by distance from the source and this should be noted.
- Exposure dose is the radiant energy delivered per unit area of a given surface in a given exposure time and is expressed in joules per square centimeter, or exposure dose = irradiance × exposure time.

Measurement in photobiology has recently been undergoing change, and although medical photobiology has been slow to follow, the change will certainly occur. The alteration is that the international standard unit of surface area is the meter and not the centimeter. Thus, the conversions are $1 \text{ J}/\text{cm}^2 = 10^4 \text{ J}/\text{m}^2$ and $1 \text{ mJ}/\text{cm}^2 = 10 \text{ J}/\text{m}^2$.

INTERACTIONS OF PHOTONS AND MATTER

Photons interact with matter in a very complex manner and most of this detail is beyond the scope of this book. However, there are a few concepts that have importance in therapy.

Absorption Spectra

All molecules are characterized by a particular absorption spectrum, or put in another way, a particular molecular species can only absorb radiation of

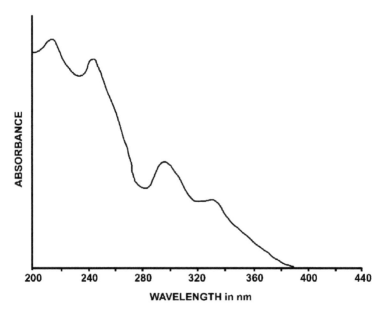

Figure 3 Absorption spectrum of 8-methoxypsoralen.

certain wavelengths. The absorption spectrum of a molecule is measured in a spectrophotometer, and since the spectrum is unique for each molecule, once it is known, it can be used for detecting the presence of that molecule. The absorption spectra of small molecules are narrow, whereas for large molecules, such as DNA, the absorption spectrum is very broad because of the variety of atoms and bonds contained within such a molecule. The absorption spectrum of 8-methoxypsoralen is moderately complex (Fig. 3).

The photobiologic effects of exposure to nonionizing radiation involve the initial essential first step of absorption of photons by some molecule, called a chromophore. Grotthus and Draper elaborated the first law of photochemistry that only absorbed radiation can cause a photochemical reaction. The practical significance of this is obvious. When radiation is being targeted at a particular chromophore, the emission spectrum of the radiation source must include the absorption spectrum of that chromophore. For example, exposure to visible radiation can never trigger the psoralen reaction, because the absorption spectrum of psoralen does not extend into the visible region.

Action Spectra

Frequently the chromophore for a photobiologic response is not known and, to aid in determining what the chromophore might be and to determine what source of radiation is most suitable for triggering the response, the

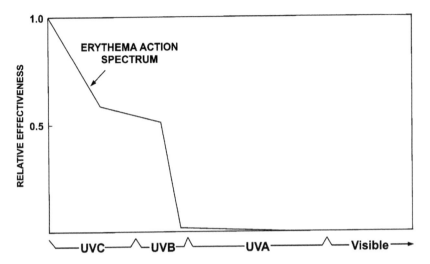

Figure 4   Action spectrum for erythema.

action spectrum for the response is measured. This is determined by testing the magnitude of the response at various wavelengths; the observations then permit construction of a curve of exposure dose of radiation as a function of the size of the response (Fig. 4). The peak of the action spectrum defines the most effective wavelengths. The action spectrum, as already mentioned, must include the absorption spectrum of the molecules. However, in biologic systems such as the skin, the action spectrum does not match the absorption spectrum of the chromophore because of the influence of the optical properties of the tissue and competitive absorption by other chromophores. The action spectrum is usually shifted to longer wavelengths, a so-called "red" shift.

Photochemisty and the Cascade

Once a photon has been absorbed by a molecule, the photon ceases to exist and all its energy is transferred to the molecule, which is now said to be in an excited state. This absorbed energy can initiate a photochemical reaction in two ways. The molecule can react with another molecule as, for example, psoralen reacts with DNA, to form a monoadduct or cross-link. Alternatively, the energy can be transferred to another bystander molecule, which in turn can interact photochemically with a third molecule; a common example of this type of reaction is the formation of excited oxygen species that react with membrane proteins.

When a photochemical reaction has occurred, a chain reaction begins involving damage to cells, release of mediators, and altered function of tissues to produce a given biologic response. Important steps in this cascade

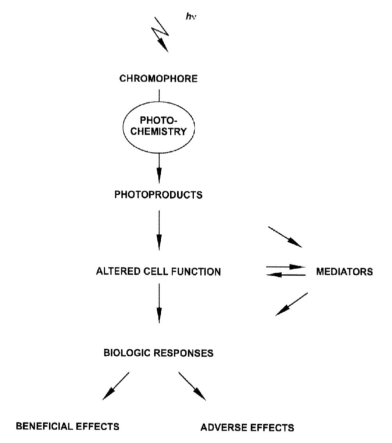

Figure 5   Possible sequence of events following exposure to nonionizing radiation (hν) leading to beneficial or adverse effects.

are the repair systems that are activated to correct the damage and prevent cell death.

It is important to keep in mind two key points: first, photobiologic responses are very complex (Fig. 5) and second, most are only minimally understood. For example, erythema and pigmentation are common biologic responses but there is only incomplete information about the steps from chromophore to altered cell function involved in producing these responses.

The Concept of Reciprocity

Reciprocity of time and dose rates is an important concept in photobiology and photomedicine. Briefly, reciprocity means that the observed effect depends only on the total dose of radiation and is independent of the duration of exposure or irradiance of the source. For example, if $100 \, \text{mJ}/\text{cm}^2$ of UVB radiation is required to produce erythema in a normal subject, then, if reciprocity holds for this response, erythema will be seen irrespective of whether the radiator produces an irradiance of $0.1 \, \text{mW}/\text{cm}^2$ ($1000 \, \text{sec}$ exposure) or $100 \, \text{mW}/\text{cm}^2$ ($1 \, \text{sec}$ exposure). For most responses in human skin, reciprocity appears to hold over many log scales. However, it cannot be assumed that reciprocity always holds and it must be tested for any given biologic response.

Thermal Effects of Radiation

Closely intertwined with the concept of reciprocity is consideration of the thermal vs. photochemical effects of radiation. Photochemical effects are specific, while thermal effects are nonspecific and do not obey the reciprocity relationship. For example, a source of radiation producing $35 \, \text{mW}/\text{cm}^2$ of UVA-2 radiation will induce photochemistry that is evident as erythema and tanning in human skin. Some heat will be generated and may make a minor contribution to the pathology, but most alterations are due to photochemical reactions. However, exposure of skin to a radiator producing $200 \, \text{mW}/\text{cm}^2$ of UVA-2 radiation will induce quite different changes. The available chromophore molecules are saturated by high photon density so that much of the energy is converted to heat, which destroys tissue. The changes observed are nonspecific ulceration and repair.

The distinction between photochemical and thermal effects is important because of the introduction of lasers into photomedicine. Most phototherapy depends on photochemistry. In contrast, photothermolysis with lasers, although it may depend on specific absorption by certain molecules, produces its effect through thermal and mechanical changes and different laws of physics are involved.

2

Sources of Nonionizing Radiation

INTRODUCTION

The sun was the first source of nonionizing radiation used in photomedicine and it continues to be used in some centers because sunlight is cheap and, in some places, abundant year-round. However, artificial sources have largely replaced sunlight due to greater flexibility.

The characteristics of a radiation source are defined by its spectral energy distribution or the more commonly used but somewhat inexact term "the emission spectrum." This describes the range of wavelengths and relative amounts of each wavelength emitted by the source. An emission spectrum may be continuous and have a smooth curve, or discontinuous and consist of a series of emission lines. There are some other terms used to describe an emission spectrum: a monochromatic source emits only one wavelength as, for example, with a laser; in contrast, a polychromatic source emits many wavelengths. Deviating into jargon, polychromatic sources are often divided into narrow- and broadband, terms which have obvious meaning if lacking a clear definition.

Determination of the emission spectrum of a radiation source requires use of a spectroradiometer, which is an expensive and sophisticated piece of equipment. Such measurements are only done in research institutions and in industry and are quite unnecessary when practicing photomedicine. However, it does no harm to know what an emission spectrum should look like. Figure 1A shows a diagrammatic representation of the emission spectrum of

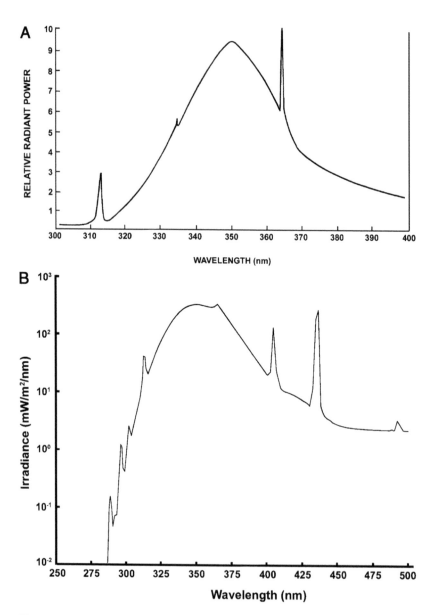

Figure 1 (A) Diagrammatic representation of emission spectrum of a Sylvania PUVA Lifeline bulb. (B) Actual measurement of emission spectrum of a PUVA bulb.

a psoralen plus ultraviolet A (PUVA) bulb provided by a manufacturer (Sylvania, Danvers, MA) and Figure 1B illustrates the actual measurements of the emission of the same bulb. It is obvious that use of a linear scale and a free-hand approach provides quite a different picture than that provided by computerized counting of photons and a log scale.

THE SUN

Solar radiation has been used as a source of UVB radiation for phototherapy and UVA radiation for photochemotherapy for centuries, but it has some distinct disadvantages.

The obvious disadvantages are that it cannot be turned on and off, it is only available at certain times of the day and the year, and insects and peeking neighbors can be a problem. The less obvious but more important disadvantage is that its biologically relevant emission spectrum varies considerably with the time of day and season of the year. The emission spectrum of the sun, as measured at the earth's surface is illustrated in Figure 2.

The main change in the spectrum of sunlight with the time of day and season of the year is in its UVB content and there are two reasons for this variation. First, UVB is absorbed by stratospheric ozone. Second, shorter wavelengths are scattered more and absorbed by more molecules than longer wavelengths. The greater the thickness of atmospheric molecules to be traversed by sunlight, as illustrated in Figure 3, the greater the chance for the shorter wavelengths to be scattered and absorbed. The shorter wavelengths also have the most energy or biologic effectiveness so it follows that in temperate climates early morning, late afternoon, and winter sunlight are not very erythemogenic or melanogenic (Fig. 4).

The shorter wavelengths of UVA radiation are also influenced to a significant degree by these seasonal and diurnal variations but the longer

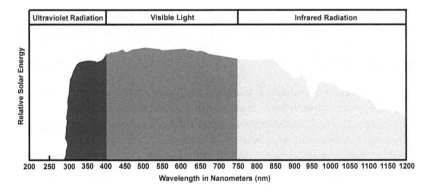

Figure 2 Emission spectrum of sun at the surface of the earth.

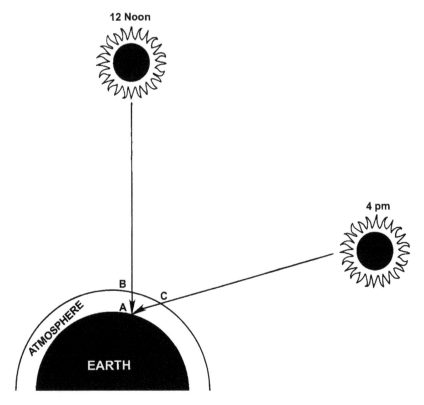

Figure 3 The distance through the atmosphere that has to be transversed by a photon is greater at 4 p.m. than at noon or A–C is longer than A–B.

wavelengths of UVA and visible light are less affected. These considerations are important because at 4 p.m. outdoors in February in Boston it is possible to develop psoralen phototoxicity in the skin but impossible for a normal person to develop a UVB-induced erythema.

FLUORESCENT LAMPS

A fluorescent lamp is essentially a low-pressure mercury vapor lamp, or germicidal lamp, with an envelope coated with a fluorescent chemical that is called a phosphor. Thus, it consists of a glass tube containing mercury vapor at low pressure, a filament as a source of electrons, and a phosphor as the lining of the tube. Electrons generated by the filament excite mercury atoms causing them to emit photons, which in turn excite the phosphor to emit fluorescent radiation of longer wavelengths. The emission spectrum of the lamp is a function of the chemical composition of the phosphor; since the

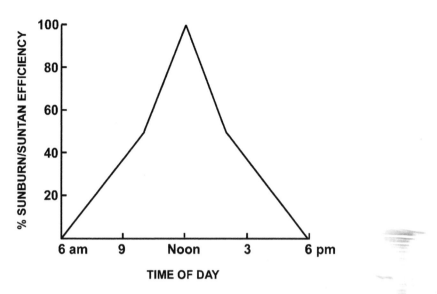

Figure 4 The effect of time of day on biologic effectiveness of UV radiation.

number of phosphors available is large, it is possible to produce a whole variety of spectra in the UV and visible regions.

Fluorescent lamps are the most frequently used source of nonionizing radiation and the mainstay of therapy because they possess a number of distinct advantages:

- Low cost of usually only a few dollars
- Reliability and a long lifetime
- Capacity to irradiate large areas
- Reasonable uniformity of radiant power with distance so that a bank of bulbs can provide much the same irradiance at points 2 in or 2 ft away
- Continuous emission spectrum so that within a given spectrum all wavelengths are represented
- High radiant power relative to heat output so that elaborate cooling arrangements are not necessary
- Inherent capacity to "tailor-make" a spectrum to suit the required purpose by using different phosphors or combinations of phosphors.

However, it is also important to recognize that fluorescent lamps do have some disadvantages and these have practical implications:

- There is variable initial output during the first few minutes after a lamp is switched on so that a lamp should be allowed to stabilize for 5–10 min before measuring the irradiance.

- Lamps are sensitive to ambient temperature, and a high temperature due, for example, to inadequate ventilation, lowers the radiant power and can alter the emission spectrum.
- The terminal 6–12 in of a fluorescent lamp has a much lower output than the center, and this can be important in treating areas such as the hands and the feet. Short lamps will have a low output unless special measures are taken to boost the output to useful levels.
- The maximal radiant power of a fluorescent lamp is limited and this can be important with UVA-1 phototherapy since large doses of this waveband are required to produce biologic effects.

HIGH-PRESSURE MERCURY VAPOR LAMP

A favorite lamp for phototherapy until quite recently was a high-pressure mercury vapor lamp, which is also called a "hot quartz" lamp or Hanovia Alpine lamp. The principle advantage of this source is a very high output of UVB radiation so that a minimal erythema dose can be delivered

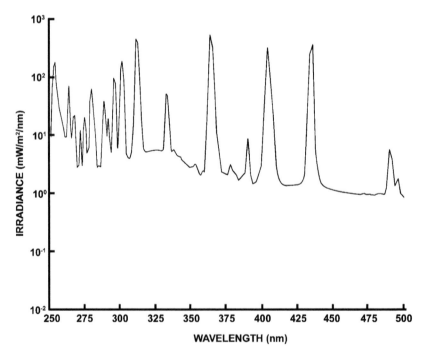

Figure 5 Emission spectrum of a Hanovia Alpine high-pressure mercury vapor lamp.

in less than a minute. However, it does have several marked disadvantages. It has a high output of infrared radiation and heat so that good ventilation is required and it cannot be held too close to the skin. Because it is operating at a high pressure, a warm-up time of 10 min or so is required to produce a stable output. The emission spectrum is discontinuous with most of the erythemally effective output at 297 nm (Fig. 5). The size of the field that can be irradiated is limited and therefore about six exposures are required for whole-body treatment. Finally, there is usually a lack of uniformity of irradiance over the entire field so that some areas are undertreated and some are overtreated. Despite these problems, these lamps are still used by some practitioners for treatment of localized disease using suberythemal doses.

METAL HALIDE LAMPS

A source of nonionizing radiation that has become popular for tanning, and to a lesser extent for therapy, is the so-called metal halide lamp. This is a high-pressure mercury vapor lamp to which various metal halides are added. Using iron, nickel, and cobalt halides, an almost continuous spectrum across UVA and UVB can be produced and the resultant output in the UVA region can be three to six times that of a fluorescent lamp. Filters can be used to isolate the UVA waveband or, alternatively, the filters can be removed to provide a good source of UVB radiation. The main disadvantages of these lamps are a high initial cost, a short lifespan, and often a small field size.

WOOD'S LAMP

An essential item in the diagnostic armamentarium of any therapist should be a Wood's lamp for help in diagnosing and delineating disorders of pigmentation. This is a high-pressure mercury vapor lamp with a nickel oxide phosphor providing a peak emission at 365 nm. The lamp is only suitable for diagnosis because of its limited spectrum, low output, and small field size.

OPTICAL FILTERS

The emission spectrum of a radiation source can be modified by insertion of optical filters that delete certain wavelengths. In therapy, cutoff filters that remove shorter wavelengths are most commonly encountered. Window glass and Mylar (a plastic) are two effective filters for eliminating wavelengths shorter than 320 nm, while various types of cellulose acetate can be used to remove wavelengths in the shorter UVB range. There are three important practical considerations in the use of filters. First, the transmittance of a filter is a curve, and thus the cutoff has a slope and is not vertical. Second,

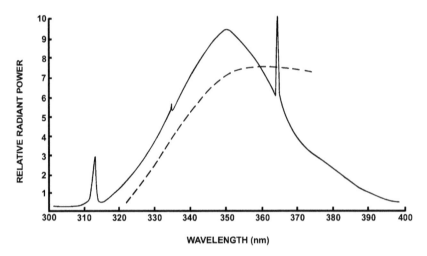

Figure 6 Effect of a cutoff filter (- - - - -) on the emission spectrum of a PUVA lamp. Note the slope of the cutoff and reduction of irradiance at longer wavelengths in the UVA waveband.

filters always eliminate a proportion of the desired wavelengths so that, for example, with a Mylar filter, there is usually a 30–40% loss of UVA radiation with the elimination of UVB radiation. These two considerations are illustrated in Figure 6. Third, filters often age or "solarize" owing to photochemical alterations induced by the incident radiation; these alterations change the transmission of the filter and hence the emission spectrum of the filtered source of radiation. Fortunately, the shift is usually to longer and hence biologically less active wavelengths.

3

Nonionizing Radiation and the Skin

SKIN OPTICS

Normal Skin

There are two important considerations regarding the optical properties of skin. First, skin optics are very complex due to the presence of a wide variety of absorbing molecules and the large number of optical surfaces available to influence the path of photons. Nucleic acids and proteins absorb the shorter wavelengths of UV radiation while melanin, a complex polymer, absorbs across the UV and visible wavebands almost like a neutral density filter. The epidermis and stratum corneum contain numerous optical surfaces. Second, the optics of skin are constantly changing as, for example, when the blood flow is increased in response to a rise in temperature, or tanning occurs following exposure to UV radiation.

When radiation strikes the skin there are four potential pathways for a photon to follow, as illustrated in Figure 1.

1. *Remission*: The photon can be reflected back from the surface or deeper layers.
2. *Absorption*: The photon can be absorbed by various chromophore molecules in any layer.
3. *Scattering*: The photon can be scattered through any layer.

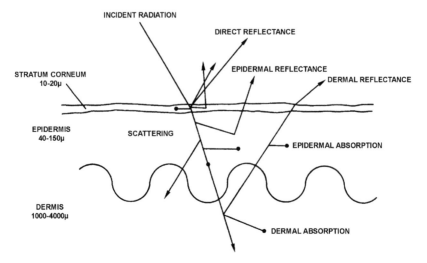

Figure 1 Possible pathways for reflectance, absorption, and scattering of photons incident on the skin.

4. *Transmission*: The photon can be transmitted inwardly to successive layers of cells until the energy of the incident beam has been dissipated.

Diseased Skin

The optics of skin can be greatly altered in the presence of a disease. Loss of melanin, as in vitiligo, decreases absorption in the epidermis resulting in increased sensitivity to UV radiation and a lowered threshold for erythema. Atrophic conditions can have a similar effect due to a loss of reflective surfaces in the epidermis. Hyperpigmentation and hyperkeratosis can have the opposite effects. Thick plaques of psoriasis are almost totally white because they reflect most visible light. Similarly, they reflect most UV radiation and thus are resistant to phototherapy.

Manipulation

The optical properties of skin can be altered for therapeutic advantage. The simplest example is application of a lubricant to scaly skin as in phototherapy of psoriasis. The oil or other lubricant fills the spaces between the layers of scale, reducing reflection and increasing transmission of UV radiation. Thinning of the epidermis by prior treatment with a retinoid or methotrexate before starting a course of phototherapy can also improve the efficacy of the treatment.

Depth of Penetration

The depth of penetration of radiation is very dependent on wavelengths. There are two main reasons for this: scattering occurs at all levels in the skin and is most pronounced for shorter wavelengths; nucleic acids and proteins absorb mainly in the UVC and shorter UVB wavebands, so that there are many chromophore molecules available in skin for these photons. The energy/depth penetration profile for UV and visible radiation is illustrated in Figure 2. In a fair-skinned Caucasian, about 15% of UVB radiation and 50% of UVA radiation reach the dermis. It is easy to remember that penetration of nonionizing radiation through skin is proportional to wavelength since we have all observed the longer wavelengths of red light being transmitted through the hand when a flashlight is placed against the palm, all the shorter wavelengths having been scattered or absorbed within the tissues of the hand.

Photon Energy vs. Penetration

The energy/penetration profile of nonionizing radiation is important in phototherapy and deserves highlighting. The energy, and hence biological activity, of a photon is inversely proportional to wavelengths as illustrated in Figure 2. Thus, UVC radiation is much more energetic than UVB radiation, a property that might suggest its usefulness in therapy. However, most of the incident UVC radiation is absorbed in the dead stratum corneum and fails to reach targets in the lower epidermis and dermis. Consequently, despite being less biologically active, UVB radiation is more efficacious for treating, for example, psoriasis, since it can penetrate more deeply and UVB photons have enough energy to activate target molecules in the dermis and epidermis. Similar considerations apply when treating psoriasis or eczema of the palms and the soles. At these sites the thick stratum corneum blocks the transmission of UVB radiation, so that this waveband is not effective in clearing disease. However, UVA radiation can penetrate this barrier, but, presumably due to the low energy of its photons, it is only mildly effective as a therapy. When a photosensitizer such as psoralen is added to the system, the therapy does become effective because then both energy requirements and the necessary penetration are satisfied.

Skin Color

Variations in skin color are due to differences in the pattern of remittance of visible radiation. Pigmented skin is dark because melanin absorbs evenly and very efficiently over the whole visible spectrum. Nonmelanized skin appears white because of high remittance over the visible spectrum. Redness of the skin is due to the increased hemoglobin content of the dermis.

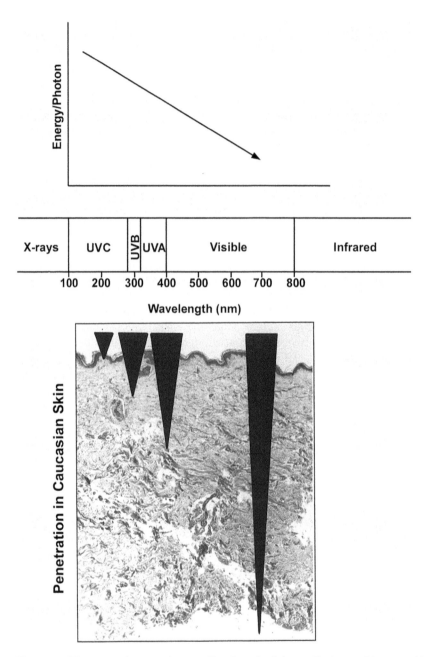

Figure 2 The energy/penetration profile of nonionizing radiation and human skin.

Hemoglobin absorbs strongly in the blue and green regions, and therefore there is a relatively larger remittance of red radiation.

MORPHOLOGIC RESPONSES TO RADIATION

Erythema

Erythema is a reflection of the vascular response to UV radiation and is often biphasic. Immediate erythema is a faint reddening of the skin, beginning shortly after the start of the exposure and fading within 30 min of the end of the exposure. Delayed erythema appears after a latency interval of 2–6 hr, peaks at 12–16 hr, and subsides over the next few days. An increase in vascular permeability accompanies both phases, and is seen as edema following a large exposure, or blistering following an even larger exposure. As commonly used, the term "sunburn erythema" denotes delayed erythema, and, unless otherwise stated, this discussion refers to delayed erythema.

The pathogenesis of erythema is poorly understood. Two main mechanisms have been proposed: the "diffusion mechanism" in which small molecular weight substances are released from damaged keratinocytes and diffuse into the dermis to act on blood vessels and the "direct-hit" mechanism in which radiation acts directly on the endothelial cells of dermal blood vessels. Possibly both mechanisms operate, either separately at different wavelengths or together, to induce different phases of erythema. The initial phase of UVB-induced erythema appears to involve prostaglandins and histamine, and there is some evidence that the later phase, after 24 hr, may involve polymorphs. This recent knowledge of the mechanism underlying UVB-induced erythema has not helped very much with treatment. Prostaglandin synthetase inhibitors, such as indomethacin, only partially block UVB-induced erythema, and antihistamines do not have any effect. Contrary to popular belief, corticosteroids, either topically or orally, also have no effect on erythema. The degree of erythema is usually evaluated semiquantitatively using the grading scale listed in Table 1. It is very important

Table 1 Grades of Erythema

Abbreviation	Description
0	No reaction
±	Faint erythema, indefinite borders
+	Minimal erythema dose, pink
2+	Red erythema
3+	Fiery red with edema
4+	Violaceous with vesiculation

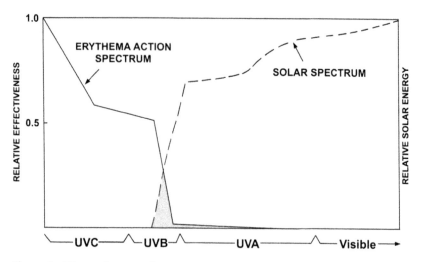

Figure 3 The erythema action spectrum.

to always refer to UV-induced erythema as "erythema" and not as a "burn" since it is readily translated into the classification of thermal burns, i.e., first-, second-, and third-degree burns. Thermal burns scar, whereas erythema is a self-healing process.

Many factors influence the development of erythema and a few important ones will be considered.

The Wavelength of Radiation

The UVB waveband is the most biologically active portion of the solar spectrum, and that waveband is responsible for most of the erythema seen following exposure to sunlight (Fig. 3). However, UVA radiation also contributes to this response. Although UVB radiation is about 1000 times more biologically active than UVA radiation, there is much more UVA radiation in sunlight. When considering broadband sources of radiation, such as a fluorescent bulb or sunlight, the possibility of interactions between the effects of different wavebands must also be considered. Unfortunately, there has been very little study of these possible interactions.

Dose

In addition to considering the absolute dose, it is important to consider the nature of the dose–response curve for a given event. For example, the dose–response curve for UVC-induced erythema is relatively flat, so that increasing the dose of UVC radiation by a factor of 10 times that required to produce erythema will not produce an increase in the intensity of the erythema (Fig. 4). A 10-fold increase in the dose of UVB above the

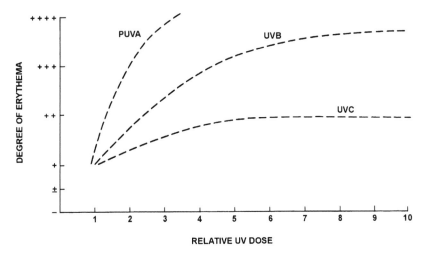

Figure 4 Dose–response curves for erythema.

erythema threshold will result in blistering. A 10-fold increase above the threshold for PUVA-induced erythema could result in a very sick patient because the dose–response curve for this reaction is steep. Alterations in dose may also change the time course of the response. For example, very high doses of radiation produce erythema that appears later and lasts longer than erythema from lower doses.

Individual Susceptibility

The presence or absence of pigmentation obviously influences the response of skin to radiation. However, for a given skin color, there is still a great deal of individual variation in the threshold of the erythemal response. The factors that determine such variation are largely unknown. The presence of photosensitizing agents such as drugs, dietary constituents, and topically applied substances must always be considered when evaluating normal, or possibly abnormal, responses to radiation.

Prior Exposure to Radiation

An important axiom in photomedicine is that the skin never forgets. Although at the end of winter the back skin and buttock skin of a fair-skinned adult may appear to be the same white color, the buttock skin and breast skin in women, if never previously exposed to radiation, will have a significantly lower threshold response to UV radiation. Thus, in an untreated patient, the skin of the perineum, buttocks, and breasts are especially prone to develop erythema.

Body Site

The body can be roughly divided into three regions with respect to sensitivity of the skin to UV radiation. The trunk, neck, and head are more sensitive, i.e., will develop erythema at a lower dose, than the upper limbs, which in turn are more sensitive than the lower limbs. The responsiveness of disease at these various sites appears to parallel the differences in erythemal responses. Thus, larger doses of radiation are tolerated by the lower limbs than by the trunk, and, similarly, larger doses are required on the lower limbs to effectively treat skin disease.

Field Size

A small area of skin requires a lower dose of radiation to develop erythema than does a large area. This is important in therapy because a dose of UVB radiation that produces erythema in a 2 cm × 2 cm test site usually will not produce erythema following whole-body exposure. Two to three times the erythemal dose is required to produce erythema for a small area over large areas of the body.

Environment

Increases in the environmental temperature and humidity, as well as wind, have been shown to decrease the threshold of sensitivity to UV radiation in mice. It is a reasonable assumption that these factors influence human responses.

Pigmentation

Background pigmentation of skin, also termed constitutive pigmentation, is the natural color of the skin and is best evaluated on nonexposed skin of the buttocks. Pigmentation resulting from external influences such as exposure to UV radiation is termed facultative pigmentation. The melanocytic response to UV radiation is also biphasic. Immediate pigment darkening is seen mainly with UVA radiation in individuals with existing pigmentation. It occurs within minutes of exposure and fades within an hour. Movement of melanosomes out of melanocytes into keratinocytes, and possibly also photochemical alteration of melanin, appears to mediate this biological response. Delayed pigmentation, which is usually referred to as a suntan, involves production of new melanin and appears within days of exposure and lasts weeks or months.

Several factors influence the development of pigmentation and a few are considered.

The Wavelength of Radiation

The action spectrum for pigmentation following exposure to sunlight (Fig. 5) is similar to the erythema action spectrum in that UVB radiation

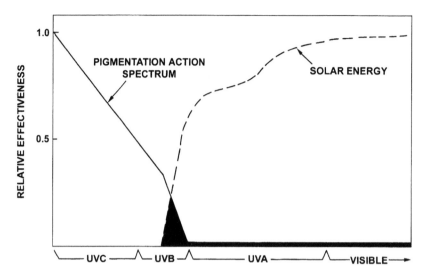

Figure 5   The pigmentation action spectrum.

is the most effective but otherwise there are significant differences. Erythemogenic doses of UVB radiation are required to produce significant pigmentation. In contrast, suberythemogenic doses of UVA radiation are very effective in inducing pigmentation. Put another way, UVA radiation can produce a tan without inducing much inflammation. In addition, visible radiation in large doses can induce pigmentation.

Constitutive Pigmentation

People with darker skin in general have a greater pigmentary response following exposure to sunlight. However, there is a great deal of individual variation. This particularly applies to people with light skin in whom it is often very difficult to predict the potential facultative response.

Age

Tanning response often diminishes with age in people with fair skin. At its most extreme are people who had an excellent tanning response in childhood and early adult life, and have minimal or no response in later adult years. This is important to bear in mind when using historical skin types in older adults.

Skin Thickening

UV exposure causes epidermal hyperplasia, and the associated thickening of the stratum corneum is a major defense against further UV damage. Even in the absence of melanization, as, for example, in an albino, thickening of the stratum corneum can lead to a 5–10-fold increase in tolerance to UVB radiation. Epidermal hyperplasia varies with wavelengths, so that for a given erythemal response, the hyperplasia is most marked following exposure to UVC radiation, less marked after exposure to UVB, and minimal after exposure to UVA radiation.

DEFINITIONS

A number of terms are used to describe cutaneous responses to radiation that have different meanings for different people, and therefore require definition.

Phototoxicity

In its broadest context, phototoxicity refers to photon-induced damage to cells or tissues and this may be evident by histologic examination only or expressed also on clinical examination. The term is used clinically in two ways. First, when a photosensitizing chemical in combination with nonionizing radiation produces a sunburn-type reaction in the skin, this is referred to as phototoxic response. The reaction is due to direct damage to the skin; it does not involve the immune system and can be produced in all people. Second, phototoxicity is often used to describe the morphologic and symptomatic evidence of acute changes in the skin, i.e., erythema, edema, and pruritus, following exposure to UV radiation alone.

Photoallergy

This is a state of specifically altered reactivity to an exogenous chemical in which photons play some role. It is an idiosyncratic reaction and mediated by a delayed hypersensitivity mechanism manifested in the skin as eczema. All known photosensitizing chemicals can produce both phototoxicity and photoallergy, but usually one reaction predominates. For example, psoralens are potent phototoxins and rarely produce photoallergy, while tetrachlorsalicylanilide is a potent photoallergen and a weak phototoxin.

Photosensitivity

This is a term used to describe a state of heightened reactivity to photons, and this may be due to photoallergy, phototoxicity, or an unknown mechanism. The term is most often used when the mechanism underlying the abnormal reaction is unknown. Hence, a patient who readily develops erythema when exposed to UV radiation is often referred to as being photosensitive.

Photodynamic Reaction

This is a term describing a phototoxic response that requires oxygen. Most photosensitizing chemicals produce their effect via excited states of oxygen that induce damage to cells; some biologists thus equate photosensitization with photodynamic reactions. The notable exceptions to this concept are psoralens and various photosensitizing drugs that feature prominently in photomedicine, since these agents can directly interact with cells and molecules without involving oxygen.

4

Nonionizing Radiation and Other Organs

INTRODUCTION

The extracutaneous effects of nonionizing radiation constitute an area of expanding interest. The eye is an obvious target for radiation-induced alterations, and both acute and chronic changes are observed. Nonionizing radiation can also alter the function of the immune, endocrine, and nervous systems. Most people have been accustomed to thinking of exposure to such radiation as a local modality with its effects limited to the skin, whereas in reality it is a systemic modality.

THE EYE

The optical properties of the eye vary with wavelength as different wavebands are absorbed in the various media of the eye (Fig. 1). UVB radiation up to 310 nm is mainly absorbed in the conjunctiva and cornea, while UVA radiation is absorbed by the lens. In a child, some UVA radiation is transmitted through the lens and reaches the retina, but in a normal adult, presumably due to photochemical changes causing a decreased transmittance in the lens, all wavelengths shorter than 400 nm are absorbed prior to reaching the retina. Fortunately, repair mechanisms in the retina are more efficient in children than in adults, and are able to deal with the insult of exposure to UVA radiation. Visible light is transmitted through the ocular tissues and absorbed by the retina so that images of the environment

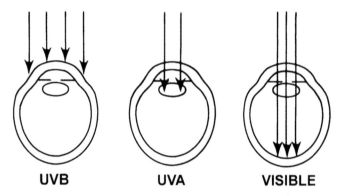

Figure 1 The absorption, and hence penetration, of radiation in the eye varies with wavelength.

may be formed. Infrared radiation also reaches the retina but does not stimulate vision.

Radiation-Induced Disorders

The site of absorption in the eye of any given waveband of radiation is usually the site of pathology produced by acute or chronic exposure to that particular waveband.

Photokeratitis

This disorder is an acute inflammation in the corneal epithelium, plus associated conjunctivitis, caused by exposure to UVB or UVC radiation. It is literally a sunburn of the eyes and follows a similar time course to the reaction in the skin. Symptoms begin a few hours after exposure and consist of grittiness of the eyes, photophobia, tearing, and blepharospasm. Corneal pain can be intense. These symptoms subside over 24–48 hr and recovery is usually complete.

Cataracts

This term refers to any loss of transmission of light by the lens, but clinically it is usually reserved for opaque lesions in the lens causing a symptomatic loss of vision. UVA radiation is absorbed by the fibers that compose the lens, and these fibers lack a repair system for removing any photoproducts that are formed. There has been much debate over whether chronic environmental exposure to UV radiation is responsible for the so-called senile cataract. Recent epidemiologic and experimental studies support this possibility, which has obvious public health implications.

Retinal Lesions

Both acute and chronic exposures to light can impair function. Exposure to bright sunlight, for example, at the beach without sunglasses, for as little as an hour or so can result in a detectable loss of vision and dark adaptation. Lifeguards have been found to lose 50% of visual capacity after 2 days of exposure to the sun without sunglasses, and this defect can persist for days or weeks.

Observation of a solar eclipse can produce permanent destruction of the cones in the fovea by infrared radiation. Laser radiation also can produce blindness, and this is due to a combination of thermal and mechanical disruption of the retina. Finally, chronic exposure to bright sunlight may be responsible for senile macular degeneration, which is a leading cause of blindness in the elderly.

Eye Protection

Fortunately, we have a number of protective mechanisms that protect our eyes from photon-induced damage. Most of the eye is embedded in the cranium, and, in addition, the corneal epithelium reflects much of the light applied to the eye tangentially. Thus, only light directly impinging on the front of the eye tends to be transmitted into the eye. The pupillary reflex also protects the eye from exposure to bright visible light since constriction of the pupil is triggered by visible radiation. However, it is important to note that the protection provided by this reflex can be nullified in two circumstances: use of sunglasses that absorb visible but not UV radiation, which is a characteristic of some commercial sunglasses, and exposure to UVA radiation sources that have a minimal output in the visible spectrum. Finally, the squinting and aversion reflexes provide some protection against intense sources of light.

Manufacturers of sunglasses have paid much more attention to fashion than health. Thus, many sunglasses can be classified as distinctly hazardous to the health of eyes, and although this is changing, there is still room for improvement. Many sunglasses have optical windows in the UV and infrared regions that permit transmission of those wavelengths into the eye. As mentioned previously, by abolishing pupillary constriction, such glasses can greatly increase the exposure dose of radiation to the lens and retina. Furthermore, even if the label on sunglasses indicates some restriction of UV transmission, it does not necessarily mean zero transmission; it should because there is no reason to permit UV radiation to enter the eye.

Many thousands of people each year have their lenses removed for treatment of cataracts, and this represents a special situation for protection of the eye against the harmful effects of radiation. The removal of the lens permits exposure of the retina to UVA radiation. A lens implant opaque to this waveband will provide protection but otherwise UV-opaque sunglasses should be used.

THE IMMUNE SYSTEM

Dramatic progress has occurred in recent years in our knowledge of cutaneous biology, and central to this progress has been the realization that the skin is an important component of the immune system. Much of our knowledge in this area has stemmed from studying the effects of UV radiation on the immune system, a research field that has coined the term "photoimmunology." A detailed elaboration of our knowledge in this area is beyond the scope of this book, but a few points important for the therapist will be outlined.

The Skin as an Immune Organ

Several components of the skin are directly involved in immune function. Langerhans' cells in the epidermis are of macrophage-monocyte lineage and function as antigen-presenting cells. There is evidence that a population of lymphocytes is normally resident in the skin.

Lymphocytes, monocytes, antibodies, and other components of the blood percolate through the vessels of the dermis, and the entire blood volume passes through the skin about every 10 min. Thus, important components of the immune system are within the range of environmental and therapeutic exposure to UV radiation. This only refers to the potential direct effects of radiation, and in the course of time we are likely to find that the indirect effects are even more important. For example, mediators released from keratinocytes or cells in the dermis following exposure to UV radiation can have distant systemic effects on the immune system. Modifications of the antigenicity of molecules, as, for example, with UV-altered DNA, might be important in disease processes. It is quite possible that some of the beneficial effects of UV radiation therapy are due to alterations of immune function, and there is certainly the potential for selective manipulation of immunity for therapeutic benefit.

Skin Cancer and the Immune System

A UV-induced alteration in immune function plays a central role in the development of nonmelanoma skin cancer in mice. Exposure to small doses of UV radiation induces the generation of suppressor T-lymphocytes that specifically block the function of a normal immunosurveillance system, which prevents the growth of UV-induced skin cancers in this experimental model. A very important question is whether similar UV-induced alterations in immune function are involved in the development of skin cancer in humans. At present the answer is maybe. An increased risk of sun-induced skin cancer in immunosuppressed patients and immune defects in patients with xeroderma pigmentosum suggest the possibility, but direct proof is as yet unavailable.

UV-Induced Immunosuppression

Most UV-induced alterations of immune function are suppressive in nature, and this has led to some people equating UV radiation with other immunosuppressive agents. This concept is quite wrong and can be very misleading for a therapist. Most immunosuppressive agents cause pan-immunosuppression so that all immune responses are affected, at least to some extent, and consequently atypical infections and systemic malignancy are often undesirable consequences. In contrast, exposure to UV radiation produces highly selective immune suppression so that some immune responses are affected while others are left completely intact. For example, UVB radiation suppresses the induction of contact allergy in the skin, but has no effect on its elicitation so that memory responses remain intact. Suppression of the induction of contact allergy, delayed hypersensitivity in the skin, and suppression of immune surveillance against skin cancer are three effects of UV radiation on the immune system.

THE NEUROENDOCRINE SYSTEM

Light and the absence of light have a marked effect on many bodily functions. Light reaching the retina activates a neural pathway to the pineal gland, which regulates production of substances that influence the functions of the brain and endocrine organs. The hormone melatonin is one product of the pineal gland, and has been the most investigated because it is readily assayed in blood and urine. Secretion of melatonin is maximal in the dark and is suppressed by exposure to bright light. Melatonin may induce sleep and may be important in controlling mood. The retina-pineal pathway entrains circadian rhythms to the light/dark phases of our 24 hr day, a fact that we are made aware of in this age of jet travel and consequent jet lag.

Exposure to UVB radiation stimulates the formation of previtamin D_3 from 7-dehydrocholesterol in the skin, then the previtamin isomerizes to vitamin D_3 under the influence of heat. Vitamin D_3, after activation in the kidney, functions to control calcium homeostatis by regulating the absorption of this mineral from the intestine. Excessive exposure to UVB radiation does not cause vitamin D intoxication because of the presence of a shutoff mechanism in skin that converts previtamin D_3 to inactive metabolites.

5

Phototesting

INTRODUCTION

Phototesting is simply a determination of a patient's level of reactivity or sensitivity to a given waveband or wavebands of radiation. The most common end point is the development of delayed erythema but sometimes other end points may be used such as development of a rash, immediate erythema, or pigmentation. Phototesting is an essential component of safe and effective delivery of phototherapy and photochemotherapy but unfortunately, many practitioners skip this step to the detriment of overall patient care.

Why Do Phototesting?

Phototesting provides a modicum of accuracy to treatment and helps solve problems associated with treatment. When starting phototherapy you can guess the starting dose but in order to avoid a symptomatic erythema, the guess is usually conservative. The result: unnecessary treatments or, worse, failed treatment due to development of excess pigmentation. When a patient develops pruritus or a rash during treatment, one possible cause is phototoxicity. Splitting the patient, covering one side while continuing treatment on the other side will give the answer after two or three treatments, since if it is phototoxicity, the treated side will be worse and the untreated side will have improved.

Why Not Do Phototesting?

There are several reasons why phototesting is not a routine procedure. It is too complicated. This is wrong. Using the simple approach outlined here any office can provide basic phototesting. It requires special equipment and training. Also wrong, since the equipment is already in the office and the training required is minimal. It is too time consuming. Yes, phototesting takes time but most insurance plans reimburse for the procedure so it provides an additional source of revenue.

INDICATIONS FOR PHOTOTESTING

Determination of the Minimal Erythema Dose

The minimal erythema dose (MED) is the most common end point used for evaluating the response of individuals to UV radiation. It is defined as the least exposure dose for a small area of skin, at a specified wavelength, that will elicit a delayed erythema response with four distinct borders, as observed at 24 hr. The observation time of 24 hr is for convenience as it is usually not the time of the maximal erythemal response.

The most important points in recording an MED are to note the site on the body where the measurement was done and the waveband used for the test. The latter is usually denoted by a subscript such as MED_{UVB} or MED_{UVA}.

Determination of the Minimum Phototoxic Dose

The minimum phototoxic dose (MPD) is often used as a guide to selecting a starting dose in PUVA therapy. It is defined as the least exposure dose for a small area of skin administered 1 hr after ingestion of 0.4 mg/kg of methoxsalen, which will produce a pink erythema with four distinct borders, as observed at 48, 72, or 96 hr after exposure. Recent studies suggest that readings at 72 and 96 hr provide a more accurate value.

Diagnosis of Phototoxicity

Development of pruritus or the sudden appearance of a psoriasiform eruption during PUVA or UVB phototherapy may signify that the patient is being overtreated and has phototoxicity. Covering half of the body and continuing treatment on the other side can rapidly confirm or refute the diagnosis.

Determination of the Minimal Urticarial Dose

The minimal urticarial dose (MUD) is an essential guide to selecting a starting dose in the treatment of solar urticaria. It is the least exposure dose required to produce urticaria within minutes of exposure of small areas of skin to the waveband selected for treatment. Obviously, if a routine schedule of treatment is used and the starting dose exceeds the MUD, the patient is likely to develop a whole-body hive with hypotension and potentially disastrous consequences.

Investigation of Photosensitivity

Patients with a history of abnormal reactions to sunlight or indoor sources of radiation can be investigated by exposure to UVB, UVA, and visible radiation in the office or by controlled exposure to sunlight.

EQUIPMENT

Four indoor sources of radiation are required for phototesting and these are available, or can be easily made available, in any office.

Broadband UVB Radiation

The bank of lamps in half of a UVB treatment unit or the four UVB bulbs in one bank of a UVA/UVB treatment unit provide a suitable source of broadband UVB radiation. Only one bank or half of the unit should be activated so as to reduce problems of shielding from stray radiation. If the unit is equipped with an internal photometer, the bank with the detector must be used.

Narrowband UVB Radiation

The bank of lamps in half of a narrowband UVB treatment unit provides a suitable source of this wavelength. The same considerations apply as outlined above in that only one bank should be activated and it should be the bank with the detector.

UVA Radiation

Half of a PUVA treatment unit is a suitable source for this wavelength and the bank used must be the one with the detector if the unit is equipped with an internal photometer.

Visible Light

A Kodak Carousel or Caramate slide projector provides a reasonably clean and intense source of visible light. An area about 10 cm × 5 cm on the ventral surface of the forearm is exposed to this source of radiation for 45 min. Any immediate or delayed reaction to this exposure is abnormal.

A Word of Warning

Small-area units and spot sources of radiation are available from some suppliers of treatment equipment and phototesting is often a suggested use for these units. If available, these units are useful for phototesting to UVA and UVB radiation since this avoids using a treatment unit which could otherwise be used for therapy. However, two strong points of caution: if treatment decisions are being made on the basis of the phototesting, the emission spectrum of the area unit must be the same as that of the treatment unit and accurate radiometry is required so as to safely transfer the results of phototesting in the area unit to the treatment unit. For example, if an MED or MPD is determined using an area unit, the area unit must have the same type of bulbs as are being used in the treatment unit. In addition, the irradiance of the area unit must be determined to arrive at a correct dose for the treatment unit.

METHODS

Determination of the Minimum Erythemal Dose

The aim of this test is to expose eight small areas to a range of doses of UVB radiation and then examine the response 18–24 hr later. A suitable size for each area is about $3 \, cm \times 3 \, cm$ square and the eight squares can be made as a template cut out of cardboard or, alternatively, an elasticized template can be purchased from equipment suppliers. The site of testing is important and should always be on the torso. The upper back is convenient but if the patient is tanned, lower back or buttock skin is suitable. The MED should not be determined on a limb since it will be higher than it is on the trunk. For example, the MED on the forearm can be twice the MED on the back and using such a reading for a treatment dose could result in marked erythema on the torso.

The selection of exposure doses is based on the skin type of the individual, the aim being to use a range centered on the anticipated MED. Some examples of suitable doses for broadband and narrowband UVB are given in Table 1, but these doses should be used only as a guide until an individual set of doses is determined by the therapist. When using a unit equipped with

Table 1 Dose Ranges of UVB Radiation for Determining MED

Skin types	Broadband (mJ/cm^2)	Narrowband (mJ/cm^2)
I–II	10–80	130–1080
III–IV	40–110	270–2160
V–VI	70–140	540–4320

an internal photometer, an easy approach is to enter the highest dose to be delivered, start the unit, then stop the unit as each dose is reached so squares can be consecutively covered. The response to these exposures is evaluated 18–24 hr later, the MED being the lowest dose that produces pink erythema with four distinct borders.

A key element in performing an MED test is effective shielding of all skin apart from the eight exposed squares. Skin that is not adequately shielded may develop a significant erythema. One approach is to use gowns, the patient's own clothing and a pillowcase over the head. A preferable quick and simple approach is to use a cloak with an attached hood made of thick fabric with a cutout in the back corresponding to the template. The cloak is then affixed to the template using duct tape. Providing a stool for the patient to sit in front of the bank of bulbs ensures lack of movement as well as some comfort during the procedure.

Determination of the Minimum Phototoxic Dose

The procedure for this test is very similar to the procedure used for determining the MED. The main differences are: the patient ingests methoxsalen in a dose of 0.4 mg/kg 1 hr before exposure, the exposure is to UVA radiation, and the results are evaluated 48–96 hr later. The range of doses selected for this test is determined on the basis of the skin type of the individual; suggested doses are given in Table 2.

Diagnosis of Phototoxicity

When a diagnosis of phototoxicity is suspected, splitting the patient can rapidly provide an answer. If the reaction is widespread, a gown can be fixed to the center of the chest and back using duct tape. Alternatively, one lower limb or a hand can be covered during treatment for more localized reactions. Treatment is continued for the other side and changes in the two sides are evaluated after two or three treatments. A clear difference usually emerges in this time, allowing a distinction between phototoxicity or exacerbation of the underlying disease.

Table 2 Dose Ranges of UVA Radiation for Determining MPD

Skin type	Dose range (J/cm^2)
I	1–8
II–IV	2–16
V–VI	10–24

Table 3 Dose Ranges of UVA Radiation for Determining MED

Skin type	Dose range (J/cm^2)
I–II	10–80
III–IV	40–110
V–VI	70–140

Determination of the Minimal Urticarial Dose

Solar urticaria affects all areas of the body and is not site specific. Therefore, testing can be done on the back prior to initiation of treatment with either PUVA therapy or narrowband UVB phototherapy. The range of doses is the same as that used for skin type I for determination of an MPD or MED and eight small squares are exposed. Urticaria usually appears within minutes but the period of observation is determined by the history given by the patient.

Investigation of Photosensitivity

In a phototherapy center, photosensitivity may arise as a consideration in a variety of circumstances. First, the patient may be referred for treatment of photosensitivity and phototesting is required to confirm the diagnosis and determine the likely response. Second, photosensitivity may be suspected from the history at the time of initial evaluation of another condition. Finally, it might arise during a course of treatment as a separate problem or because of photoexacerbation of the underlying disease. The approach to investigation varies mainly according to the suspected diagnosis.

Polymorphous light eruption is best confirmed by an exposure to sunlight since it will produce a positive response in almost all patients. Testing using indoor sources of radiation produces a much lower response rate. The patient is instructed to expose a previously affected area to a sufficient dose of sunlight. For example, if by history the arms are involved and 30 min of noonday sun usually produces the reaction, one arm can be exposed for this period and if the response is positive, the patient then comes to the office for inspection of the rash and possibly a biopsy.

For other forms of photosensitivity suitable investigation is determination of the MED_{UVB}, MED_{UVA} and a single exposure to visible light. Suitable doses for determination of a MED_{UVA} are listed in Table 3. The evaluation of the responses depends to some extent on the suspected diagnosis. Solar urticaria gives an immediate response, usually within minutes. All patients should be evaluated at 24 hr to determine and record the MED reactions. In patients with lupus, photoexacerbated psoriasis and chronic actinic dermatitis, a rash may be delayed for 2–3 weeks.

Management of Psoriasis Vulgaris

Psoriasis vulgaris is the disease most frequently treated with phototherapy and photochemotherapy, and the duration of experience with these treatments is longest in this disease. Phototherapy with UV radiation has been a standard treatment for psoriasis vulgaris for decades, while PUVA therapy has been used for the past 30 years. Therefore, psoriasis vulgaris will be used as the prototype disease for a practical discussion of the approach to both treatments. These treatments are only one aspect of the overall management of psoriasis and are seldom used as the sole therapy. Thus, this section will aim to place the treatments in the context of the total therapy of the patient with psoriasis vulgaris.

Many patients present a very negative attitude toward treatment of their disease because of past disappointments. The aim of the therapist is to replace this negativism with a positive attitude that the disease can be successfully treated. The initial, and often the most important, step in changing the attitude of the patient is the first consultation, which must contain several key elements, as outlined in Table 1. First, the patient and the disease require a full evaluation so that the physician knows the patient and the patient's environment, the nature of the disease, and how the patient feels about the disease. Second, it is essential to explain that psoriasis is a chronic disease, that there is no quick fix or cure, but that there are some very successful treatments that can control psoriasis in most patients. Third, the patient must be educated about all possible treatments; a handout is a valuable addition but not a substitute for this explanation. Fourth, the treatment

Table 1   Essential Elements of Initial Consultation

Evaluation of the patient and the disease
Explanation of the nature of psoriasis
Discussion about possible treatments
Tailoring the treatment program to the patient
Selling the treatment

---

program outlined to the patient must be tailored to the patient and the disease. The treatment must have a reasonable risk/benefit ratio, be effective for the type of disease being treated, and be within any financial, social, or geographic constraints of the patient's situation. Finally, the patient must not only agree with the treatment program but must also be "sold" on the treatment or it will not be used.

This initial consultation takes time, and for the patient with moderate-to-severe psoriasis who is a candidate for UV or systemic therapy, at least 30 min is required, while if a combination treatment is suggested, the visit will take about 45 min. However, it is time well spent because for most patients it will be the last extended consultation required for a long time.

6

Evaluation of the Patient

INTRODUCTION

When PUVA therapy, UVB phototherapy, or systemic therapy is being considered as part of the management, a careful evaluation is particularly important because these are often long-term treatments that are time consuming for the patient and associated with certain risks. Thus, the evaluation should aim at determining the suitability of the treatment for the patient and the suitability of the patient for the treatment and should also assess the likely risk/benefit ratio of the treatment. Careful documentation is also important, and evaluation forms should be used to ensure that no important aspects have been forgotten. Such a form is best compiled to suit the needs of the individual physician or clinic, but the content should include all the points discussed here.

THE PATIENT

Age

PUVA therapy and systemic therapy are relatively contraindicated in children. Fortunately, few children have severe psoriasis, but occasionally, when the disease is disabling, consideration must be given to using UV therapy with a strong preference for phototherapy.

Sex

Caution must be exercised in women of reproductive age when considering PUVA therapy or systemic agents. While on PUVA therapy, women should be instructed to practice birth control and if a woman becomes pregnant, PUVA therapy should usually be stopped. Psoralens have not been associated with birth defects and UVA photons do not penetrate to the uterus so that pregnancy is a relative contraindication to PUVA therapy. Phototherapy is the preferred treatment during pregnancy.

Skin Phototype

Phototherapy is usually the treatment of choice in patients with skin types I and II because of the long-term risks of photoaging and skin cancer from PUVA therapy in these patients. In contrast, skin types IV–VI are better treated with PUVA or combination treatment since they are likely to fail phototherapy due to excessive tanning and long-term risks are negligible.

Motivation and Competency

The motivation of the patient should be explored, because unless a patient is strongly motivated, treatment is likely to be unsuccessful. An assessment of intelligence is also necessary, because PUVA therapy is somewhat complex and mistakes are likely to occur with illiterate and unintelligent patients.

THE DISEASE

Extent

Guidelines for PUVA therapy usually emphasize that more than a certain percentage (usually 30%), as determined by the rule of nines of the body surface, must be involved by disease before this treatment is considered. This approach is not only arbitrary but also misleading, because, although the extent of disease is a factor to consider, it is certainly not the only one. For example, 20% involvement limited to exposed areas in a 20-year-old patient is likely to be more disconcerting for the patient than is 60% involvement limited to covered areas in an 85-year-old patient. Furthermore, it is often difficult to decide on the extent of the disease. Do coin-sized lesions that involve all areas of the body but with large amounts of intervening normal skin represent 100% involvement? Obviously not, but the patient often considers this to be whole-body involvement. However, it must be emphasized that minimal disease is not an indication for UV therapy.

Site

The site of involvement is usually very important. Disease limited to exposed areas is much more troublesome to the patient than disease restricted to covered areas. The site of the disease is also important to the therapist. If the disease is limited largely to the scalp and intertriginous area, i.e., the regions that receive the least exposure to radiation, UV treatment is less likely to be successful. Facial involvement should always raise the possibility of photosensitive psoriasis. Involvement of the palms and soles usually indicates a requirement for PUVA therapy since phototherapy is not effective at those sites. The exception to this rule is young children in whom phototherapy may be effective.

Type of Lesions

Thick lesions, particularly if there is a lot of scale, and inflammatory psoriasis favor the use of PUVA therapy, combination treatment, or a systemic agent. Thin, macular psoriasis is likely to respond to phototherapy.

Associated Symptoms and Arthritis

Associated symptoms such as pruritis should be evaluated because these are part of the disability caused by the disease. The presence and severity of associated arthritis are important, because methotrexate or a biologic agent may be a better option than PUVA therapy in patients with severe arthritis.

Effect of Sun Exposure

Most patients find that psoriasis is improved by sun exposure, but a few find the condition exacerbated, and these latter patients tend to do poorly with UV therapy.

Disability

When all the elements of the disease have been evaluated, it should be possible to make an assessment of the degree of disability that the patient experiences as a result of having psoriasis. Disability is difficult to quantify, but it is one of the main factors to consider in assessing whether a patient requires an aggressive approach to therapy. A patient should be significantly disabled by psoriasis before UVB phototherapy is considered. The treatment is time consuming and expensive and requires good motivation for a successful result. This requirement for significant disability applies even more to PUVA therapy and systemic agents because of the long-term hazards of the treatments.

PREVIOUS TREATMENT FOR PSORIASIS

Information about previous treatment that the patient has received is valuable for assessing how much disability is caused by the disease, the possible therapeutic options available, and the likely response to and risks of the therapy. A poor response to other treatments suggests that the patient is left with few options. A failed response to UVB phototherapy argues in favor of trying PUVA therapy, but exacerbation by UVB phototherapy may suggest that failure with PUVA therapy is likely to occur. Past exposure to ionizing radiation or arsenic for the treatment of psoriasis and large exposures to UVB phototherapy or sunlight are warnings that the risk of skin cancer will be increased with PUVA therapy.

PAST AND CONCURRENT CONDITIONS

Medical History

A history of, or symptoms suggestive of, a connective tissue disease should be sought. Other relative contraindications such as renal and hepatic disease should be noted. UV therapy is stressful for the patient and therefore general infirmity and severe cardiovascular disease are relative contraindications since the patient must stand for the duration of the treatment.

Immunosuppression, as in organ transplant patients and human immunedeficiency virus (HIV) infection, should be noted. Cardiac transplant patients and to a lesser extent renal transplant patients have a greatly increased risk of skin cancer so that UV therapy is relatively contraindicated. An increased risk of skin cancer has not been documented in HIV-infected patients but this may emerge as the duration of survival increases.

Drug History

Exposure to UVA radiation as in PUVA therapy can photoactivate medications and trigger a photoallergic or phototoxic response. Systemic photoallergic reactions are so rare that this possibility can be ignored. Systemic phototoxicity can be of clinical significance with a few drugs: doxycycline, demeclocycline, amiodarone, and the quinolone group of antibiotics. If a patient is on these drugs the starting or continuing dose of UVA radiation should be reduced by 25%. Many other drugs, including the thiazide diuretics and most of the nonsteroidal anti-inflammatory agents, are labeled as being photosensitizers but in practice rarely cause a problem, so their use should be noted but no other action is required.

Dermatologic History

Patients must be asked about a personal or family history of melanoma and a personal history of removal of nevi, actinic keratoses, or skin cancer.

SOCIAL AND ECONOMIC FACTORS

The life-style and economic status of the patient are often the main factors in determining whether a therapy is suitable. UV treatment requires a large time investment by the patient and is usually an office therapy. These factors can also guide the decision of using PUVA therapy vs. UVB phototherapy. PUVA therapy is effective when given twice weekly and requires infrequent maintenance, whereas UVB phototherapy usually requires three treatments a week and at least weekly maintenance treatment.

Geography

Patients living a long distance from a treatment center are usually not candidates for UV therapy.

Occupation

Patients who have heavy work schedules or travel a lot will have poor compliance. Deep-sea fishermen and traveling salesmen are poor candidates for UV therapy. Furthermore, occupation plays a role in determining disability. For example, cosmetic appearance can be of central importance in occupations involving a lot of contact with the public so that psoriasis on exposed areas can be a major disability.

Financial Cost

UV therapy is expensive relative to topical therapy but inexpensive as compared to biologic agents. Insurance coverage is often a deciding factor in determining selection of treatment.

PHYSICAL EXAMINATION

A whole-body skin examination is essential before considering PUVA or UVB therapy. The nature and extent of psoriasis must be determined, but in addition the patient should be carefully examined for melanomas, suspicious-looking nevi, keratoses, and nonmelanoma skin cancer. Any suspicious lesion should be biopsied. An assessment of existing solar damage should also be made. Freckling, telangiectasia, wrinkling, and diffuse hyperkeratosis on exposed skin should be noted. Nonexposed skin of the buttock should also be examined, as this area is a guide to the development of premature aging of the skin during long-term therapy.

LABORATORY INVESTIGATIONS

No laboratory investigations are required prior to the initiation of either UVB or PUVA therapy, unless dictated by other health concerns raised by the history and examination of the patient. Although more extensive initial and follow-up investigation for PUVA patients was originally suggested, long-term observation of patients has found that laboratory parameters are not adversely affected by this treatment.

If the history or clinical examination is suggestive of an associated connective tissue disease, a lupus package of tests should be ordered and it is sometimes useful to enlist the aid of a rheumatologist or internist if unexplained findings require further investigation. Similarly, if significant renal or hepatic dysfunction is suspected, it should be investigated before initiating PUVA therapy.

OPHTHALMOLOGIC EXAMINATION

At the time of initiation of PUVA therapy, all patients must have a complete eye examination performed by an ophthalmologist. In an ideal world this examination would be obtained prior to the start of therapy but since this might result in much delay and the ocular complications of PUVA therapy are a long-term hazard, arranging for the examination within a few weeks is a satisfactory compromise. Similarly, if a patient has had a normal eye examination in the past few months this would be acceptable provided it is documented. The examination should include a slit-lamp examination of the lens and cornea, funduscopic examination of the retina, and determination of visual acuity. The examination should be repeated yearly, or more often if abnormalities are found.

BIBLIOGRAPHY

Drake LA, Ceilley RI, Dorner W, Goltz RW, Graham GF, Lewis CW, Salasche SJ, Turner MLC, Lowery BJ. Academy guidelines. Guidelines of care for phototherapy and photochemotherapy. J Am Acad Dermatol 1994; 31:643–648.

Stern RS, Kleinerman RA, Parrish JA, Fitzpatrick TB, Bleich HL. Phototoxic reactions to photoactive drugs in patients treated with PUVA. Arch Dermatol 1980; 116:1269–1271.

Stern RS, Morison WL, Thibodeau LA, Kleinerman RA, Parrish JA, Geer DE, Fitzpatrick TB. Antinuclear antibodies and oral methoxsalen photochemotherapy (PUVA) for psoriasis. Arch Dermatol 1979; 115:1320–1324.

Stern RS, Lange R. Outcomes of pregnancies among women and partners of men with a history of exposure to methoxsalen photochemotherapy (PUVA) for the treatment of psoriasis. Arch Dermatol 1991; 127:347–350.

7

The Therapies Available

INTRODUCTION

Treatment modalities with antipsoriatic activity can be broadly divided into three groups: topical, UV radiation, and systemic. This sequence also roughly defines their risk/benefit ratios: topical agents are usually the safest and of benefit only in limited disease, while systemic agents carry the greatest potential risk and should be used only in extensive disease. During the initial consultation with a new patient, each of these treatment options should be explained and an evaluation given as to their application and limitations in the particular case. The patient's confidence in his or her physician will be somewhat dampened if he or she reads the next day in the *New York Times* about some new treatment that is the latest and greatest therapy for psoriasis and it was not even mentioned.

TOPICAL AGENTS

The most commonly used treatments for psoriasis are topical agents. Many patients with mild disease use over-the-counter agents that claim antipsoriatic activity or simple emollients and never consult a physician. Those who do consult a physician are likely to be given a prescription for a corticosteroid, calcipotriene (Dovonex®), or, most recently tazarotene (Tazorac®).

The advantages and disadvantages of topical therapy are listed in Table 1. Perhaps the greatest disadvantage of all the available topical agents

Table 1 Advantages and Disadvantages of Topical Therapy

Advantages
  Ease of use at home
  Low cost
  Quick effect
  Low risk of side effects
Disadvantages
  Messy and unpleasant to use
  Improves but does not clear the disease
  Decreased effect with time

is that they rarely if ever convert psoriasis to normal skin. However, despite this limitation most physicians agree that they are the best agent for treating mild disease and they are useful as adjunctive treatment for patients on UV therapy.

UV RADIATION

The sun has probably been used in the treatment of psoriasis for as long as the disease has existed, since most patients know that they improve during the summer or a winter vacation in the tropics, and it can be used as an effective and popular treatment in selected patients. However, an important limitation of sunlight as a therapy is that it usually improves rather than clears psoriasis; this may be due to its limited availability or the lack of a controlled approach to the treatment. In comparison, exposure to artificial sources of UV radiation can rapidly and consistently clear psoriasis.

Therapeutic exposure to UV radiation has some advantages over topical therapy and perhaps the main advantage is that it can convert psoriasis to skin that is morphologically and histologically normal. The advantages and disadvantages are listed in Table 2. In most patients with moderate-to-severe

Table 2 Advantages and Disadvantages of UV Therapy

Advantages
  Cosmetically acceptable treatment
  Clears disease in most patients
  Maintenance provided
  Long-term remissions
Disadvantages
  Office procedure
  Time consuming
  Expensive
  Adverse effects
  Intertriginous areas/scalp not treated

psoriasis UV therapy is the treatment of choice because of a high response rate, it can maintain patients in a controlled state and, when used as an intermittent treatment, it can produce long-term remissions.

SYSTEMIC THERAPY

The most significant recent change in therapy of psoriasis has been the rapidly expanding selection of systemic agents. Twenty years ago there was only one truly effective agent, namely, methotrexate, and now there are seven approved drugs and still counting.

Methotrexate

This is a very effective agent for treatment of moderate-to-severe psoriasis since it has a high clearance rate and can provide long-term control of the disease. Depression of the bone marrow is the main short-term problem with methotrexate. The main long-term problem is impairment of liver function, and this occurs in 25–40% of the patients. Methotrexate is teratogenic and therefore should not be used in women of child-bearing age without adequate contraception during treatment and for 1 month after cessation of the drug. Another problem is that methotrexate appears to alter the nature of psoriasis, making it a more aggressive disease. Thus, a person may have had the ordinary plaque type of psoriasis but after receiving methotrexate for several years may develop unstable, inflammatory psoriasis when an attempt is made to shift to another treatment. The guidelines for methotrexate therapy have been published. Several different regimens are used, but the approach of dividing the weekly dose into three doses given at consecutive 12 hr intervals appears to be the most effective and safest.

Retinoids

Acitretin is the preferred drug for the treatment of psoriasis because isotretinoin is less effective. The main indications for acitretin are the erythrodermic and generalized pustular types of psoriasis, and in a daily dosage of 0.6–1 mg/kg of body weight, this drug is equally as effective as methotrexate in the treatment of these two rare forms of the disease. Acitretin is not very useful as a sole agent in the treatment of the ordinary plaque type of psoriasis; in some patients the disease is partially controlled, but to achieve complete clearance, months of therapy are required. The major disadvantage of long-term acitretin therapy is that it produces side effects in 100% of the patients. The most common adverse effects involve the skin and mucous membranes, and these are inconvenient rather than hazardous. However, hyperlipidemia, liver abnormalities, and calcification of tendons occur in 50–85% of the patients. The long-term significance of some of these side effects is still unknown, and thus use of the drug should be restricted to the rare patient who is unresponsive to other less hazardous therapy. Acitretin is markedly teratogenic and should not be used in any women of child-bearing age.

Cyclosporine

This is an agent with limited usefulness in treatment of psoriasis because of the risk of nephrotoxicity. However, it does produce rapid clearance in most patients and good short-term control so it is useful as a salvage therapy in a person with severe disease and few options.

Biologic Agents

Recently a number of immunomodulatory drugs have been approved for treatment of moderate-to-severe psoriasis and psoriatic arthritis. These agents are given by self-administered subcutaneous injection, intramuscular injection, or intravenous infusion. The response rates in psoriasis vary from low to very high while short-term problems have been minimal. The long-term adverse effects of these agents are not known.

OTHER ASPECTS OF TREATMENT

Reduction of Trauma

Trauma to the skin is a significant factor in inducing psoriasis, as evidenced by the Koebner phenomenon and localization of the disease to certain areas such as the elbows and knees. Telling patients to reduce the amount of trauma to the skin is good advice, but, except in specific instances, it is not a practical approach to treatment. Use of a condom in a person with psoriasis of the penis and protection of the hands, if they are affected, are two specific examples.

Reduction of Stress

Emotional stress is also a trigger for psoriasis, but, again, telling patients to reduce the amount of stress in their lives is easy rather than practical advice. The use of meditation exercises during PUVA and UVB therapy does increase response rates in terms of the number of patients cleared and treatments required for clearance. Certainly, there are some patients who suffer a flare-up of disease whenever the social milieu becomes stormy. However, there are many other patients who go through deaths, divorces, operations, and other stressful experiences without fluctuation of the disease or the need for increased treatment to control the disease. Alcohol abuse is an issue that has been raised in psoriatic patients. Anecdotal comments have claimed that alcohol exacerbates psoriasis, but there is no evidence to support this. It is possible that patients drink because they have severe psoriasis rather than vice versa, if indeed they do consume more alcohol than other people.

Centers treating a large number of patients with psoriasis can provide a support-group structure that is very useful for some patients. Feelings of stigmatization, concern about the success of treatment, and the long-term prognosis of the disease can be aired in small groups with considerable benefit. The groups can meet regularly under the guidance of a nurse, supplemented at times by attendance of a physician. A few patients require psychological counseling or treatment by a psychiatrist when their ability to cope with the disease or the treatment is questionable.

Monitoring of Medications

Several medications can induce or exacerbate psoriasis and should be avoided by patients if possible. Lithium and the antimalarial drugs are the main offenders. Beta-blockers can induce a psoriasiform eruption as a rare side effect, and there are a few reports of the exacerbation of existing psoriasis. The role of systemic corticosteroids in the exacerbation of psoriasis is more complex. When first exposed to these agents, usually for treatment of an unrelated inflammatory condition such as allergy to poison ivy, most patients with psoriasis have a dramatic remission of their disease. However, as the corticosteroid is withdrawn there is often an equally dramatic exacerbation.

National Psoriasis Foundation

Providing information about the National Psoriasis Foundation can be a worthwhile therapeutic measure in many patients. These patients have a desire to "do something" about finding a cause and cure for their disease, and contact with this organization provides an outlet for these feelings. Furthermore, patients feel that they are being kept up-to-date about psoriasis through information in the Foundation's newsletter.

Physicians can also benefit by being a member of this organization through its educational endeavors, referral network, insurance advocacy, and provision of leaflets for patient information.

Education of Patients

Mention has already been made about "selling" the patient on the selected treatment plan and of giving patients a clear explanation of the disease, treatment options, and the specific treatment. In addition, every patient should be given at least two pamphlets at the end of the initial consultation: one explaining the nature of psoriasis and the treatment possibilities and the other explaining the specific treatment selected for that patient. These can be generated by the physician or pamphlets available from the Psoriasis Foundation or other organizations can be used.

BIBLIOGRAPHY

Bernhard JD, Kristeller J, Kabat-Zinn J. Effectiveness of relaxation and visualization techniques as an adjunct to phototherapy and photochemotherapy of psoriasis. J Am Acad Dermatol 1988; 19(3):572–574.

Kabat-Zinn J, Wheeler E, Light T, Skillings A, Scharf MJ, Cropley TG, Hosmer D, Bernhard JD. Influence of mindfulness meditation-based stress reduction intervention on rates of skin clearing in patients with moderate to severe psoriasis undergoing phototherapy (UVB) and photochemotherapy (PUVA). Psychosom Med 1998; 60(5):625–632.

8

Which Therapy to Use?

INTRODUCTION

During the consultation with a new patient with psoriasis vulgaris the physician must produce a plan of action for treatment and this plan is based on a detailed analysis of the patient and the disease and an understanding of the likely risks and benefits of each available treatment. Psoriasis represents a continuum from the patient with minimal disability to the patient with incapacitating disability. The decisions about management of the extremes are fairly easy. The patient with a few lesions of psoriasis, so-called mild disease, is best treated with a topical agent or perhaps an excimer laser. The patient with generalized disease bordering on a pustular or erythrodermic phase will require systemic therapy, at least in the short term. The patients in the middle of the continuum will probably benefit from UV therapy. The aims of this discussion are to provide guidance first as to whether UV therapy should or should not be used and second whether the choice should be PUVA or UVB phototherapy.

INDICATIONS FOR UV THERAPY

The most common indication for UV therapy is disabling psoriasis unresponsive to topical therapy. Since the definition of disability can vary among individuals, it is best determined on a case-by-case basis as a consensus between physician and patient. It is unwise to treat minimal disease with UV therapy for two reasons. First, such treatment has a poor risk/benefit ratio. Second, UV therapy rarely achieves complete clearance: a person with 1% body involvement cleared of 95% of the disease may still be an unhappy patient. In contrast, a person with 50% body involvement who achieves 95% clearance will be delighted. UV therapy is indicated in a few patients as the initial treatment because of explosive onset of widespread psoriasis. Finally, UV therapy is indicated in some patients as they cycle off methotrexate or some other systemic therapy.

CONTRAINDICATIONS TO UV THERAPY

In certain situations, PUVA therapy, UVB phototherapy, or both treatments are contraindicated.

Absolute Contraindications

1. Xeroderma pigmentosum should not be treated with UV radiation, because patients with this disease have defective repair of UV-induced damage in DNA, which affects all cells in the body.
2. Albinism because of high risk of developing skin cancer.
3. Lupus erythematosus with a history of photosensitivity or a positive Ro antibody test.
4. Lactation is a contraindication to PUVA therapy but UVB phototherapy may be used.

Relative Contraindications

Treatment may be used with caution in the following circumstances taking into consideration the severity of the indication for treatment, alternative options for treatment, and the anticipated duration of treatment.

1. History or family history of melanoma.
2. Past history of nonmelanoma skin cancer, previous treatment with ionizing radiation or arsenic, and extensive solar damage are contraindications to PUVA therapy in most patients. The main exception to this is the older patient over 60 years of age, but this decision will depend on the need for treatment and other options available. These situations are also contraindications to UVB phototherapy on theoretical grounds, although the evidence

for this is either unavailable or weaker than it is with PUVA therapy.

3. Uremia and severe hepatic failure are usually contraindications to PUVA therapy because drug metabolism and excretion will be disturbed. However, both groups of patients can be treated with careful monitoring.
4. Pemphigus and pemphigoid are probably exacerbated by both UVA and UVB therapy.
5. Immunosuppression.
6. Pregnancy is usually a contraindication for PUVA therapy but UVB phototherapy may be used.

Certain other contraindications are sometimes raised. Cataracts and aphakia are not contraindications but rather a warning that careful attention must be paid to eye protection. Photodermatoses are also a warning, since they may be triggered or exacerbated by treatment; however, they also respond to the treatment.

PUVA THERAPY OR UVB PHOTOTHERAPY?

For the physician with access to both UVB phototherapy and PUVA therapy, the question arises as to which to use when. In making this decision four important differences between these two treatments must be kept in mind:

- PUVA therapy is more effective than UVB phototherapy in clearing psoriasis in most patients.
- PUVA therapy is a much more convenient and effective maintenance treatment.
- UVA radiation is more penetrating than UVB radiation; that is, UVA penetrates through a greater depth of tissue.
- PUVA therapy is probably associated with a greater risk of long-term adverse effects.

Factors that suggest use of UVB phototherapy include the following:

1. The disease
   - Psoriasis of recent initial onset. It is possible that long-term maintenance treatment will be unnecessary. The extreme example of this is acute guttate psoriasis, which should always initially be treated with UVB phototherapy.
   - Thin, macular psoriasis.
   - A history of rapid and easy clearance on exposure to sunlight.

- Psoriasis with a demonstrated photosensitivity to UVA but not UVB radiation.

2. The patient

   - Pregnancy, lactation, or intention to become pregnant.
   - Young age: A child with psoriasis may have a lifetime of disease ahead, and it is best to use the safest treatments first and leave more potent treatments for later.
   - Skin type I that always burns, never tans, or a past history of x-ray or arsenic treatment. These patients are prone to PUVA-induced skin cancer.
   - Illiteracy or low intelligence.
   - Patient preference for avoiding oral medications.

Factors that suggest use of PUVA therapy include the following:

1. The disease

   - A long history of psoriasis. This suggests that maintenance therapy will be an almost certain requirement.
   - Thick plaques.
   - Involvement of the palms and soles. UVB therapy is without significant effect at those sites.
   - Nail disease.
   - Psoriasis with a demonstrated photosensitivity to UVB but not UVA radiation.
   - Failure to respond to UVB phototherapy.
   - Active, aggressive disease with a marked inflammatory component. Erythrodermic and pustular psoriasis are the extreme examples of this situation.

2. The patient

   - Skin types III and higher. Pigmentation appears to be less of an obstacle to successful clearance with PUVA therapy than with UVB phototherapy.
   - Geographic, social, or occupational factors that necessitate keeping treatments to a minimum.

Most these features of the disease or the patient are relative and not absolute requirements for one treatment rather than the other. Furthermore, in addition to the factors listed, there are two other elements that will influence the decision but are not easily quantified. Some physicians will favor one treatment more than the other because they feel more "comfortable" with it. Some patients will be quite adamant in preferring one treatment, and this might be for a rational or irrational reason. For example, a common reason is that a friend or member of the family responded to a particular treatment, and therefore the patient will not be swayed from having the same treatment.

9

Oral PUVA Therapy

INTRODUCTION

The acronym PUVA was originally introduced to describe oral methoxsalen photochemotherapy or, more specifically, the combination of oral administration of methoxsalen and subsequent exposure to an artificial source of UVA radiation. The term has been broadened in common usage to include therapy with other psoralens, topical administration of the photosensitizer, and use of the sun as the source of radiation. These variations should be defined to avoid confusion, e.g., topical trisoralen PUVA therapy. This chapter is restricted mainly to a discussion of oral methoxsalen photochemotherapy, since it is the most frequently used form of the treatment, and the variations will be discussed at the end.

Psoralens are a group of phototoxic compounds that can interact with various components of cells and then absorb photons to produce photochemical reactions that alter the function of the cellular constituents. The psoralen reaction is an example of a photosensitized response in which an exogenous chromophore is introduced with the aim of altering the biological response of tissue to radiation. Much is known about the properties of psoralens and the waveband, UVA radiation, that excites these compounds, but relatively little is known about how the psoralen/UVA radiation interaction influences the function of tissue.

PSORALENS

Background and History

Psoralens belong to the furocoumarin group of compounds that are derived from the fusion of the furan ring with coumarin. The parent compound psoralen and many of its derivatives are naturally occurring compounds found in a large number of plants. The psoralen content of plants is responsible for inducing phytophotodermatitis, which is simply a phototoxic reaction in the skin manifested as varying combinations of erythema, blistering, and increased pigmentation. Psoralens are present in fruits and vegetables such as limes, lemons, figures, and parsnips or may be present in certain fungi that contaminate vegetables. Thus, psoralens are ingested in small amounts as a part of most ordinary diets and in quite significant amounts in a pure vegetarian diet. The biological significance of this fairly constant exposure to psoralens is unknown. To keep things in perspective, it would require the ingestion of several pounds of figs or parsnips to cause clinical phototoxicity with normal exposures to solar radiation.

The medicinal properties of psoralens have been known for centuries, and their use in the treatment of vitiligo was recorded as long ago as 1550 BC. Thus, PUVA therapy is hardly a new idea. Plant extracts were applied to the skin or taken orally like a cup of tea, and the patients then exposed themselves to sunlight to produce phototoxicity in the vitiliginous skin and subsequent repigmentation. In the Middle East and Asia today, similar plant extracts are still sold in the markets and used by patients in this somewhat crude form of PUVA therapy. El Mofty at the University of Cairo first used a purified psoralen for the treatment of vitiligo in 1947.

Four psoralens are used in PUVA therapy but only one of these compounds is approved for use in the United States. Methoxsalen or 8-methoxpsoralen (Fig. 1) is obtained from the seeds of a plant called *Ammi majus*. It was first introduced for treatment in America in 1951. Trioxsalen or 4,5-8-trimethylpsoralen is a synthetic compound introduced in 1964 for therapy of vitiligo but it is no longer marketed in the United States. Bergapten or 5-methoxypsoralen is available in Europe for treatment and psoralen is used in some countries for the treatment of psoriasis and vitiligo.

Pharmacology

There are several aspects of the pharmacology of methoxsalen that the therapist must keep in mind since they can have a great influence on treatment response; they are summarized in Table 1.

Absorption

Methoxsalen is poorly soluble in water and this is a limiting factor in its absorption from the gastrointestinal tract. Most studies have found that

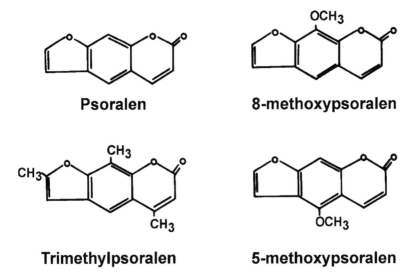

Figure 1 Psoralens used in therapy.

food, particularly fat, retards absorption and diminishes peak blood levels. There is a lot of interindividual variation in the absorption of the drug, in terms of both the amount absorbed and the rate of absorption. Peak blood levels vary a great deal and their timing also varies, consequently different patients will be on different phases of their absorption curves at the time of treatment. Therefore, it is important to treat patients at a consistent time after ingestion. As illustrated with two hypothetical examples in Figure 2, if patients A and B are treated at 2 hr after ingestion instead of 1 hr, patient A may develop marked erythema and patient B will get little benefit from the treatment. In practice, if a patient is more than 30 min late for an appointment, they should not receive a treatment on that day.

There is some intraindividual variation in the absorption of methoxsalen, and this is mainly due to what the patient has eaten and the time of day. Patients should be warned about this and urged to be consistent with both diet and the time of treatment.

Table 1 Important Features of Psoralen Pharmacology

Insolubility in water impedes absorption
Large interindividual variations in absorption
Significant but saturable first-pass effect in liver
Concentration in skin determines therapeutic effect

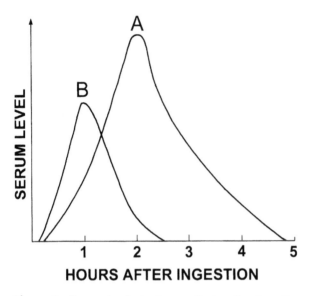

Figure 2 Serum levels in two patients after ingestion of a standard dose of methoxsalen.

First-Pass Effect

Methoxsalen is subject to a significant but saturable first-pass effect in the liver. This means that a proportion of any dose is metabolized by the liver after absorption and never reaches the skin. However, since this effect can be saturated, as the dose is raised, the proportion of active compound reaching the skin rises. For example, in an adult, 10 mg methoxsalen may produce no detectable plasma level, 20 mg may give a level of 20 ng/mL of serum, and 40 mg may give a peak level of 300 ng/mL. Since the drug is only available as 10 mg capsules, this is of utmost importance to patients taking 10 or 20 mg. A reduction in dose from 20 to 10 mg might result in a complete loss of therapeutic effect. Conversely, an increase from 10 to 20 mg, or even 20 to 30 mg, may result in erythema.

Concentration in Skin

The only concentration level that is of importance is the level at the target site in the skin since it is there that an interaction with UVA radiation will yield therapeutic benefit. The serum levels of these compounds can be measured by thin-layer chromatography, high-pressure liquid chromatography, and other techniques, but such measurements are only a guide to the absorption of psoralens. Direct measurement of the phototoxic response of skin is the only means available for assessing the cutaneous content of psoralens.

Metabolism and Excretion

After oral administration, methoxsalen is distributed to all organs of the body, but in the absence of photochemical binding excretion is rapid. The compounds are metabolized in the liver and excreted via urine, feces, and expired air. Drugs activating cytochrome P-450 enzymes enhance and accelerate metabolism of methoxsalen and hence increase the first-pass effect through the liver. Metabolism is virtually complete and little of the active compound is excreted.

Photobiology

Methoxsalen cannot photosensitize unless photons are absorbed. The absorption maxima of methoxsalen are at approximately 212, 245, 295, and 330 nm, with slight absorption extending into the longer UVA waveband. Thus, it might be expected that methoxsalen would be activated by wavelengths in the UVC or UVB regions. However, determinations of action spectra in vivo have shown that psoralen photosensitization occurs with wavelengths >320 nm. Early studies in guinea pigs and humans indicated that the action spectrum for delayed erythema with psoralens was between 340 and 380 nm. This led to the use of UVA bulbs with a peak emission at those wavelengths, and these are the bulbs still used in therapy. More recent studies suggest that maximal photosensitization occurs at the shorter wavelengths of 320–340 nm, but the precise action spectrum has not been defined. Of course, there is a slight problem in attempting to define an action spectrum for cutaneous toxicity from psoralens at wavelengths <320 nm, namely, UVB-induced erythema.

UVA RADIATION

Broadband Sources

Methoxsalen is mainly used in combination with broadband sources of UVA radiation. There are two characteristics of the emission spectra of such sources that are important in determining the magnitude and nature of the elicited response.

Emission vs. Action Spectrum

First, there is the relationship between the emission spectrum of a source and the action spectrum for the psoralen reaction in skin. The emission spectrum of the radiation source depicted in Figure 3A peaks at 350 nm and extends from 300 to 400 nm, while the action spectrum for psoralen is diagrammatically shown as having a peak at 330 nm. Thus, only radiation contained within the shaded area will be involved in the psoralen reaction. The peak of the emission spectrum of the source depicted in Figure 3B is

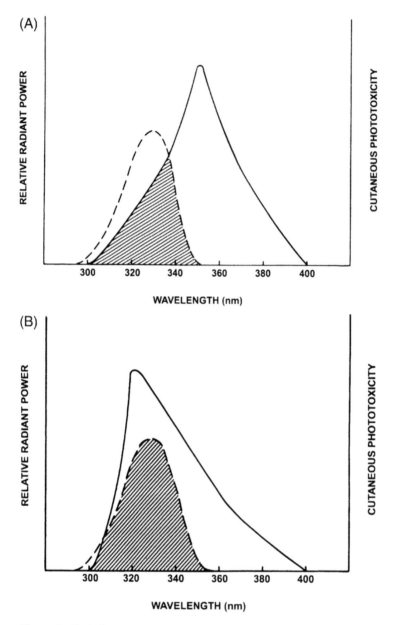

Figure 3 Emission spectra of two radiation sources for a 320–400 nm waveband. Diagrammatic representation of action spectrum for psoralen/UVA radiation (- - -). A greater proportion of action spectrum lies within the emission spectrum shown in B than in A.

quite different, even though the limits of the spectrum (300–400 nm) are the same. The amount of radiation contained within the shaded area in Figure 3B is much greater than in Figure 3A, and therefore this source would be more efficient at triggering a reaction with psoralens.

Biologically Active Wavebands

The second characteristic of the emission spectrum that must be considered is its content of other biologically active wavebands. Thus, a source that contains a significant amount of UVB radiation can be expected to produce a different cutaneous response from that produced by a pure source of UVA radiation. The effect produced by UVB radiation may be additive to or synergistic with the psoralen/UVA reaction.

From these considerations, it is obvious that the cutaneous response to psoralen/UVA radiation may vary among radiation sources that have different emission spectra. The UVA fluorescent bulbs that are available from U.S. manufacturers at present all have essentially the same emission spectrum. The point has already been made that this may not be the optimal emission spectrum for psoralen photosensitization of skin. However, when and if bulbs with different spectra are introduced, it will be necessary to redefine the cutaneous responses to psoralens before using them in treatment protocols.

Alternative Sources of Radiation

Metal Halide Lamps

Metal halide lamps with suitable filters can also be a useful source of UVA for activating psoralens. Their main advantage is a high irradiance so that treatment times are short, while their main disadvantage is cost.

Sunlight

The sun is a very convenient source of UVA radiation but is not a safe radiation source for use with methoxsalen, because the therapeutic dose with this agent is close to the phototoxic dose; therefore, severe erythema is a common problem. The high content of UVB radiation in sunlight may also contribute to this problem. Insects, prying neighbors, and seasonal variations are other problems that arise with the use of the sun as a source of UVA radiation.

Black-Light Bulbs

Standard black-light bulbs can be used as a radiation source, but owing to their low irradiance, treatment times will be long. The emission spectrum of most black-light bulbs is also different from that of PUVA bulbs in that there are a higher proportion of longer wavelengths and the psoralen reaction therefore tends to be less efficient.

Tanning Lamps

Most lamps used in tanning parlors or for home use have a peak emission in the shorter wavelength (320–340 nm) of UVA radiation and therefore are likely to be much more effective in activating psoralens as compared to PUVA bulbs. These lamps also emit a significant amount of UVB radiation and this will add to their unpredictability in psoralen activation.

CUTANEOUS RESPONSES

PUVA treatment produces erythema, pruritus, and pigmentation of normal and abnormal skin. The cutaneous responses to PUVA treatment appear to be influenced by the same factors that modify the development of UV-induced erythema. These influences, particularly prior exposure to radiation, body site, and field size, are important considerations in therapy.

Erythema

There are four features of PUVA-induced erythema that are of paramount importance:

> *Time course*: Erythema from PUVA treatment appears later and lasts longer than UVB-induced erythema. PUVA-induced erythema usually appears after 36–48 hr (Fig. 4), but in some patients it

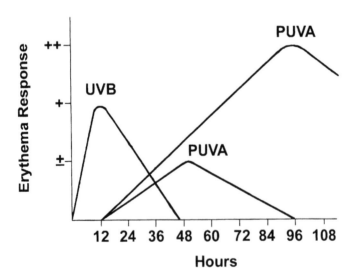

Figure 4 Time course of PUVA- and UVB-induced erythema. Note that more intense erythema peaks later.

may be delayed until 72 hr. A mild erythema will usually subside in 96 hr, but a marked erythema can persist for 2 or even 3 weeks.

Peak intensity: The more intense the erythema the later will it reach a maximum. As can be seen in Figure 3, a $\pm$ erythema and a 2+ erythema can look much the same at 48 hr and it is not possible to predict where the patient is going to be at 96 hr or even later. The take-home message is that it is extremely unwise to treat in the presence of erythema.

Dose–response curve: PUVA-induced erythema also has a steep dose–response curve (Fig. 5). Thus, the dose required to produce a 4+ erythema with blistering is only a few multiples of the dose that produces a 1+ erythema. In contrast, the dose–response curve for UVB-induced erythema is much less steep. These differences between the erythemal responses to PUVA and UV radiation are important in therapy, because small alterations of treatment frequency or UVA dosage can result in very painful erythema.

Symptoms: All UV-induced erythemas are associated with pruritus and may be painful. However, for a given level of erythema a PUVA-induced erythema is associated with much more pruritus and pain. PUVA treatment also can be associated with a deep, burning itch, a feeling like insects crawling under the skin, and this can persist for weeks or even months. This response is probably due to direct phototoxic injury of cutaneous nerves.

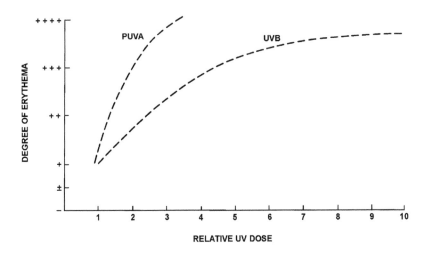

Figure 5 Dose–response curve for erythema following exposure to PUVA and UVB radiation.

Pruritus

The PUVA itch is a symptom associated with most erythemas but, in addition, it may be a symptom of phototoxicity in the absence of erythema. In the latter case, it typically begins on the outer aspects of the arms and the thighs, the buttocks, and in women on the breasts.

Pigmentation

PUVA produces pigmentation in all patients with functioning melanocytes. Pigmentation after oral administration of psoralen and exposure to UVA radiation is usually darker and lasts longer than the tan associated with comparable UVB-induced erythema. Pigmentation following topical application of psoralens and exposure to UVA radiation can last for months or years. Treatment with PUVA therapy produces hyperplasia of the epidermis and thickening of the stratum corneum. These changes, together with pigmentation, are effective in raising the threshold for erythema from subsequent exposure to UV radiation with or without psoralens.

An important consideration which is often overlooked is that pigmentation from PUVA therapy occurs both in normal skin, where it is perceived as a tan, and in plaques of psoriasis where it is disguised by the erythema. A biopsy of a psoriatic plaque in a patient with a dark tan and persistent disease reveals loads of melanin and this is often the reason for the failure to clear the disease.

CELLULAR RESPONSES

Photoactive psoralens intercalate between the bases of DNA in the absence of radiation. Absorption of photons by psoralens results in photochemical binding to a pyrimidine molecule to give a monofunctional adduct. With some compounds, including methoxsalen and trioxsalen, a second photon can be absorbed, resulting in a cross-link to a pyrimidine molecule on the sister strand of DNA. Such cross-links are also called bifunctional adducts. Cells can repair psoralen photoadducts, but cross-links are more difficult to repair than are monofunctional adducts. In turn, it is probably more difficult for a cell to repair monofunctional adducts than UVB-induced lesions in DNA. Psoralens also react with RNA, protein, and cell membranes, but the importance of these reactions is unknown.

TREATMENT SCHEDULES

Methoxsalen Dosing

Methoxsalen is available from only one pharmaceutical company in the United States: Valeant Pharmaceuticals International, Costa Mesa, CA. Two formulations are available (Table 2) but the improved liquid formulation

Table 2 Formulations of Methoxsalen

Trade names	8-MOP	Oxsoralen Ultra
Formulations	10 mg as crystals in pink capsules	10 mg as liquid in green soft gelatin capsules
Absorption	Poor and erratic	Better and more consistent
Dose	0.6 mg/kg	0.4 mg/kg

(Oxsoralen Ultra) introduced in 1987 should be used in all cases because of superior results due to better and more consistent absorption. Sometimes, pharmacists and health plans regard 8-MOP as the generic version and insist on it being used. This is incorrect as neither are generic drugs and they both cost the same per capsule; since Oxsoralen Ultra can be used in a lower dose, it is in fact cheaper. It is wise to mention to the patient that they should be given green capsules when their prescription is filled.

The dose of Oxsoralen Ultra methoxsalen is approximately 0.4 mg/kg (see Table 3) and is taken 1 hr before treatment; it is important to avoid food for 1 hr before and after ingestion. It must be noted that each of these aspects of use are at variance with the package insert, and alert patients, and sometimes pharmacists, will be quick to point out these discrepancies. Valeant recommends taking the medication with food such as milk. Most studies have found that food, particularly fat, retards absorption and diminishes peak blood levels. The company also recommends using a dose of 0.6 mg/kg, but if taken without food, the drug produces too many adverse effects at this dose. Finally, they also recommend a treatment time of 2 hr after ingestion of the medication. Most studies have found peak blood levels about 1.5 hr after ingestion, and in practice, it is much more convenient for patients to use a delay of 1 hr after ingestion.

Determination of Sensitivity to PUVA Therapy

There is marked variation in individual sensitivity to PUVA therapy, and this is mainly due to differences in constitutive and facultative pigmentation.

Table 3 Dose Schedule for Oxsoralen Ultra

Patient weight		Drug dose (mg)
(lb)	(kg)	
<66	<30	10
66–143	30–65	20
144–200	65–90	30
>200	>90	40

Sensitivity to PUVA therapy in terms of erythemal response has two aspects: threshold sensitivity to the initial dose of UVA radiation and long-term sensitivity to cumulative exposure to radiation. Both aspects of sensitivity need to be determined for any given patient, and there are two methods commonly used.

Skin Typing

The most commonly used method for assessing the likely tolerance of the patient for therapy is to assign a "skin type" (Table 4). The patient is asked about his response to a 30 min, noontime exposure to sunlight at the beginning of summer to determine skin types I through IV, while skin types V and VI are decided on the basis of examination of the skin. Many patients, particularly the elderly, are unable to readily answer the question as outlined, and follow-up questions are necessary:

> Have you ever had a sunburn?
> Do you always sunburn?
> Do you tan at all?
> Do you freckle?

It must be emphasized that skin typing is a very imprecise evaluation, subject to much observer and patient error. Several studies have found a poor correlation between skin typing and determination of the minimum phototoxic dose (MPD). However, in practice it has proven to be a satisfactory method for determining the initial and subsequent exposure doses of UVA radiation.

Determination of the MPD

The sensitivity of a patient to PUVA therapy can also be determined by measuring the MPD (see Chapter 5).

Table 4 Skin types

Skin type	History	Examination
I	Always burn, never tan	
II	Always burn, sometimes tan	
III	Sometimes burn, always tan	
IV	Never burn, always tan	
V		Brown[a]
VI		Black

[a]Chinese, Mexican, American Indian.

Which Technique Should You Use?

In the United States most people use skin typing to determine exposure doses because it is simple, less time consuming, and therapeutically successful. However, in Europe, particularly in some specialized centers, phototesting is the preferred approach. Intuitively, phototesting should be advantageous in terms of reducing the number of treatments and dose of UVA radiation required to clear psoriasis and the frequency of erythema. However, in the only prospective bilateral comparison study that compared the two approaches skin typing was superior in some aspects to the MPD method. The side of the body treated on the basis of phototesting did clear in two or three fewer treatments but the final dose and total cumulative dose of UVA radiation and the frequency of erythema were far higher on that side than on the other side treated on the basis of skin typing.

Frequency of Treatment and Doses of UVA Radiation

The dose of UVA radiation and the frequency of treatment are the two variables in PUVA therapy since the dose of methoxsalen and the interval between ingestion of the drug and exposure to UVA radiation are both fixed in any given patient.

A variety of schedules for PUVA therapy have been suggested and tested in different studies. No one schedule is ideal for every patient, but instead the therapist should use all schedules and select the correct one for the individual patient. This selection should be based on:

- The skin type of the patient
- The type of disease
- Previous and current response to treatment
- Social and geographic factors

The goal of PUVA therapy is to clear psoriasis but it is important to remember that the treatment has two constraints (Fig. 6):

- The risk of developing erythema from being too aggressive. PUVA therapy in most people's hands is a suberythemogenic treatment. There are two good reasons for this. First, it is not necessary to induce erythema in order to clear psoriasis. Second, and perhaps more important, PUVA-induced erythema of symptomatic severity is very unpleasant. It lasts for days or even weeks, is painful, and is associated with extreme pruritus. Thus, the main aim of treatment is to avoid erythema while still using effective doses of UVA radiation.
- The risk of developing too much pigmentation from being too conservative. This is of most concern with skin types III through VI.

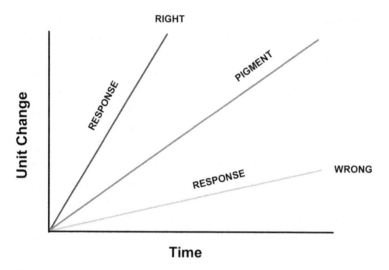

Figure 6 Potential responses to PUVA therapy in terms of clearance of disease as compared to development of pigmentation.

B.I.W. and T.I.W. Schedules

The features of a twice a week (B.I.W.) and a three times a week (T.I.W.) schedule of treatment are given in Table 5. In skin types I and II, B.I.W. and T.I.W. treatments appear to be equally efficacious in that a similar number of treatments are required to clear the disease with these two schedules; thus, one schedule (B.I.W.) just takes longer to achieve clearance. In skin types III and higher, T.I.W. treatment is more effective than B.I.W. because it permits clearance of psoriasis to proceed more rapidly and minimizes the hindrance of pigmentation.

The starting doses, the increments, and the final clearance doses of UVA radiation are determined by skin type (Table 6). Treatments are given at least 48 hr apart to allow for an assessment of the erythemal response to the preceding treatment. If there is no erythema, the dose of UVA radiation is increased each treatment until satisfactory clearance of disease has occurred. If faint erythema is present, the dose of radiation is held constant.

Table 5 B.I.W. and T.I.W. Schedules

Most widely used PUVA schedules
Treatments given 48 hr apart
Improvement usually seen between treatments 6 through 10
Average number of treatments to control psoriasis is 25–30

Table 6 Dose of UVA Radiation for B.I.W. and T.I.W. Schedules

Skin type	UVA radiation dose (J/cm^2)		
	Initial	Increments	Final
I	1.5	0.5	5
II	2.5	0.5	8
III	3.5	0.5–1.0	12
IV	4.5	1.0	14
V	5.5	1.0	16
VI	6.5	1.0–1.5	20

If definite or tender erythema is present, treatment is stopped until it has faded.

There are two groups of patients who require a different schedule: all patients with skin type I and older patients with skin type II, in particular those patients who have carefully avoided any exposure to sunlight for many years. The dose of UVA radiation should only be increased weekly in these patients at least until their erythemal sensitivity has been established, and, in addition, any evidence of erythema is an indication to withhold treatment. Furthermore, a B.I.W. rather than a T.I.W. schedule is best in these patients. These two groups of patients account for a considerable proportion of unexpected erythemas and caution should be exercised in treating them.

The final doses listed in Table 6 are intended only as a guide for the therapist. PUVA therapy is an interaction between methoxsalen in the skin and incident UVA radiation. It follows that the patient who absorbs methoxsalen very well and thus has a high skin level of drug will probably clear at a low dose of UVA radiation and vice versa.

An important point that the therapist must keep in mind and explain to the patient is that weekly (Q.W.) treatment is not a clearance schedule but rather a maintenance schedule. Patients on a B.I.W. schedule often think that Q.W. treatment will be just half as effective and become discouraged when they miss treatments and fail to improve. With a few exceptions, Q.W. treatment will hold the patient steady at a given phase of clearance and often make subsequent clearance more difficult because of excess pigmentation.

11011 Schedule

The features of this schedule are listed in Table 7. It appears to exert a very different effect on psoriasis as compared to other schedules. Fewer treatments and lower doses of radiation are required to clear the disease. The

Table 7 11011 Schedule

Treatment on four days each week: Monday, Tuesday, Thursday, Friday
UVA dose increased every third treatment: Monday and Thursday
Final clearance dose is 4–12 J/cm^2
Average number of treatments to clear is 15

---

initial dose of UVA and increments in dose are determined by the skin type
of the patient (Table 8).

The 11011 schedule should be considered for any patients of skin types
III or higher and is almost essential for skin types V and VI. In addition, it is
a partial solution to the problem of patients with asbestos-type psoriasis or
very thick plaques; combination treatment with a retinoid or methotrexate is
preferable in these patients, but if there is a contraindication to these treatments, a 11011 schedule is a reasonable compromise. The main disadvantages of this schedule are that erythema is more of a problem, particularly
in skin types I and II, and the logistics of attending a treatment center four
times a week can be a problem for any patient.

Schedule Based on MPD

The B.I.W., T.I.W., and 11011 schedules can be employed using initial and
subsequent doses of UVA radiation based on an initial determination of the
MPD and the features of this treatment are listed in Table 9. The weekly
increases are of course determined by the presence or absence of erythema.

Additional Treatments

Extra treatment of certain areas of the body should be initiated at the start
of treatment regardless of which schedule is used. These areas are:

1. Disease on the lower limbs and to a lesser extent the upper limbs
   is usually slower to clear than disease on the trunk. If there is

Table 8 Doses of UVA Radiation for 11011 Schedule

| Skin type | UVA radiation dose (J/cm^2) | |
	Initial	Increments
I	0.5	0.5
II	1.5	0.5
III	2.5	0.5
IV	3.5	1.0
V	4.5	1.0
VI	5.5	1.5

Table 9 Schedule based on MPD

Determination of MPD: read at 72 hr
Starting dose of UVA: 50–70% of MPD
Treatment given two to four times a week
Increase weekly by 30%

significant disease at these sites, an extra exposure should be given after the whole-body exposure. The patient puts on an examination gown and ties it around the buttocks, puts a pillowcase over the head to protect the face, and receives an extra exposure to the limbs.

2. Severe nail involvement or palmar and plantar psoriasis will usually require additional treatment. A hand and foot unit is best for this purpose, but if unavailable the door of a stand-up unit is a reasonable substitute.

3. Plaques around the ankles are usually very slow to respond to treatment. There is no ideal way of treating this area, but a makeshift approach that usually works is to give an extra treatment in the stand-up unit, with most of the patient's body outside. The patient sits clothed on a chair outside the unit with the exposed feet resting on a low stool or small stepladder inside the unit. The door is closed around the legs as much as possible while the additional treatment is given.

The dose for each of these extra treatments is determined by skin type. Patients with skin types I and II can be started at 1 J/cm^2 and increased by 0.5 J/cm^2 each treatment. Patients with skin type III and above can be started at 2–4 J/cm^2 and increased by 1 J/cm^2. When satisfactory clearance of all areas of the body has been achieved, most of these additional treatments can be stopped. The exception to this is the extra treatment to the limbs in a patient who had marked disease at this site; this additional treatment should be continued since the sudden drop in exposure dose is likely to lead to recurrence.

Disease in the intertriginous areas of the groin, axillae, and under the breasts can be a marked problem is some patients. The only solution, albeit one that is unavailable to most therapists, is a lie-down or bed unit in which the patient can concentrate comfortably on exposing these areas. These units are widely used in Europe but have not been generally available in the United States. Adjunctive treatment with a topical antifungal plus a mild corticosteroid cream is a useful alternative.

RESPONSE TO PUVA THERAPY

The response to PUVA therapy is outlined in Table 10.

Table 10 Response to PUVA Therapy

Skin
Improvement by treatment 6–10
Clear by treatment 30
Clear of disease = >95% of skin clear
Skin is normal or hypo-, hyperpigmented
Nails
All types of nail involvement may respond
About 50% respond
Response seen after 4–6 months of treatment
Scalp
Requires additional therapy to clear
Often stays clear on maintenance therapy
Arthritis
Probably not influenced by treatment

Disease on Exposed Skin

When a B.I.W. or T.I.W. schedule is used, some evidence of improvement in the disease is usually seen by the fifth or sixth treatment. If there is no change by the 10th treatment, the patient is a slow responder and the cause of this should be sought (see Chapter 20). Failure to achieve significant improvement by treatment 20 or clearance by treatment 30 is usually accepted as a treatment failure. In this situation another approach to treatment should be considered. In most studies, more than 90% of patients have achieved satisfactory clearance within 30 treatments.

During resolution the size of the skin lesions does not change but instead there is a gradual decrease in scaling and thickness to yield macular erythema. This then fades and usually leaves even pigmentation of the skin. Patients with skin types III through VI may be left with residual hyperpigmentation that fades over a few weeks in skin types III and IV but may persist for months in skin types V and VI. Patients with chronic plaques of long standing may develop hypopigmentation, often dotted with freckles, at these sites. A plaque of psoriasis is therefore considered to be clear when it merges with normal skin or there is an increased or decreased amount of pigmentation. Persistent erythema is either persistent psoriasis or replacement of psoriasis by phototoxicity.

Clearance of disease is usually defined as >95% of body surface free of disease. However, satisfactory clearance and control of disease will depend on the hopes and desires of the patient, and some patients will be pleased to accept <95% of body surface free of disease. The resistant areas are usually the elbows and knees, and even if these are cleared, recurrence occurs at these sites in many patients on regular maintenance treatment. Usually, very high doses of UVA radiation are required as maintenance therapy to maintain a completely disease-free state.

The duration of a remission after successful clearance with PUVA therapy is longer than with UVB phototherapy both with and without maintenance treatment. In the absence of a maintenance phase, more than 50% of patients remain clear at 6 months and more than 30% of patients are clear after 1 year.

Nail Disease

Nail disease is slow to clear on PUVA therapy, and improvement of this condition, if it occurs, will not be seen until after several months on maintenance therapy. All types of nail disease may respond to PUVA therapy, and we have observed resolution of pitting, although this has not been the finding of other studies. After 4 months of maintenance treatment, 50% of patients with nail disease had achieved resolution of this problem in one large study that we conducted.

Scalp Disease

As already noted, psoriasis of the scalp requires additional therapy if the patient has a normal amount and distribution of scalp hair. However, once disease on the scalp is controlled by topical therapy, it is often not necessary to continue such treatment. Presumably, the small amount of UVA radiation that reaches the scalp is insufficient to achieve clearance of disease but can maintain a clear state. Laser therapy using a 308 nm excimer laser is a very effective alternative to topical treatment and should be considered in any patient with resistant disease.

Psoriatic Arthritis

There is one report that psoriatic arthritis is helped by PUVA therapy, but that has not been the finding in our studies. Arthritis was unchanged after more than 6 months of PUVA therapy in one group of patients evaluated. Arthritis in large joints would require a systemic effect of PUVA therapy, as very little UVA radiation penetrates to the synovium of joints other than the small joints of the hands and feet.

MAINTENANCE THERAPY

One of the main advantages of PUVA therapy is that it is possible to maintain patients in a relatively clear state using infrequent treatment, once their disease is controlled.

Schedule

The last clearance dose of UVA radiation is held constant as the maintenance dose. Thus, the cumulative dose of radiation received during the maintenance phase of treatment is very dependent on the final clearance dose, hence the efforts during the clearance phase to keep this dose as low as possible by using aggressive schedules and combination treatments.

There is no fixed schedule for maintenance because individual responses are very variable and the schedule outlined in Table 11 should only be used as a guide.

Response to a Recurrence of Disease

If the recurrence is minor and confined to the knees and elbows or consists of a few small lesions of no great significance to the patient, treatment can be held at the current frequency or even continued to be decreased in frequency. However, a significant exacerbation of disease is a reason to halt the sequential reduction in the frequency of treatment. The possible responses in this situation hinge on the nature of the exacerbation and some of the possibilities are outlined in Figure 7. Perhaps the most important thing to note in this flowchart is that the dose of UVA radiation is never increased unless a clearance schedule is resumed. The reason for this is that an increase in dose on a maintenance schedule merely raises the tolerance of the skin without clearing the disease. When a patient is put back on a clearance schedule, the dose of UVA radiation may be raised if it is considered to be too low, but often the simple increase in frequency of treatment will suffice in regaining control of psoriasis.

How Long Should It Be Continued?

Fortunately, most patients decide this for themselves and stop coming for treatment. For those patients who continue maintenance treatment, it is essential for the physician to play an active role in determining the duration and frequency of treatment, with the aim of minimizing treatment and hence long-term adverse effects. Several factors need to be considered:

- If a patient has active disease, then continued maintenance therapy is probably necessary.

Table 11 Maintenance schedule for PUVA therapy

Four treatments at weekly intervals (Q.W.)
Then four treatments every other week (Q.2W.)
Then four treatments every third week (Q.3W.)
Then four treatments at monthly intervals (Q.M.)

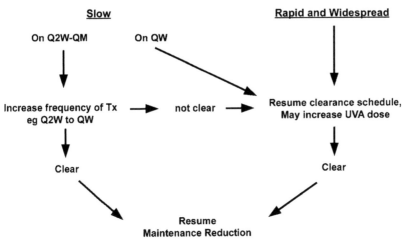

Figure 7 Algorithm for management of exacerbation of disease in the maintenance phase of treatment.

- The higher the skin type of the patient, the less concern there should be about continuing maintenance treatment.
- Maintenance treatment at a frequency of Q.2W. or Q.3W. on a long-term basis may result in less overall exposure than repeated courses of clearance treatment.

Finally, a very practical point. If the patient has had 4 months of monthly treatment without any significant recurrence, treatment can probably be stopped. However, when a patient elects to continue maintenance treatment on a monthly schedule, care must be taken that erythema does not occur as a result of progressive decrease in pigmentation. A 10% reduction of the exposure dose with each treatment after 4 months usually avoids this problem.

PRECAUTIONS

The therapist must focus attention in two directions. First, psoralens enter all cells in the body and not just those affected by the psoriatic process. Second, there is a large amount of UVA radiation in sunlight that can activate psoralens from the time of ingestion of the drug until it is excreted. Therefore, emphasis must be placed on protection of tissues that are not involved in the disease process and avoidance of inadvertent exposure to UVA radiation. The eye is the most important consideration. Methoxsalen

Table 12   Protection during PUVA therapy

During radiation
Eyes shielded by UVA-opaque goggles
Male genitalia covered with a jockstrap
Face protected
After ingestion of psoralen
Eyes protected by UVA-opaque glasses
Skin protected by clothing and sunscreens and avoidance of outdoor activities
Nontreatment days
Exposure to sunlight minimized
UV-blocking sunglasses worn

---

enters the eye and UVA radiation is absorbed by the lens. If the eyes are not protected from UVA radiation, cataracts may form after repeated phototoxic insults.

There are three points during treatment at which protection must be considered (Table 12).

During Treatment

The eyes must be shielded by UVA-opaque goggles or wrap-around glasses during treatment; most patients prefer small goggles to avoid the raccoon look. The only exception to this rule is people who have involvement of the eyelids with disease who can be trusted to keep their eyes closed during the whole treatment. Several studies have shown that the eyelids are effective barriers to UVA radiation. The male genitalia are sensitive to PUVA therapy and the incidence of skin cancer at that site is high. Therefore, provided there is no disease on the genitalia, male patients should wear a jockstrap or underpants during treatment. The face should also be shielded if it is not involved since it receives frequent exposure to UVB radiation and does not need the additional insult of PUVA therapy. Application of a sunscreen before treatment or use of a pillowcase over the head during treatment are suitable means of protecting the face.

The one potential problem of shielding any area of the body during treatment is that the patient will forget to shield the area one day and the result is severe erythema. For example, a person may have always worn a pillowcase to shield the face, but for treatment 30, when the exposure dose is 15 J/cm^2, forgets to use the pillowcase and the result is a very painful erythema on the face and neck. This is a strong argument against piecemeal treatment of the body and in favor of limiting shielding to areas such as the face and genitalia so both the staff and patient can ensure that it is always done.

After Ingestion of Psoralen

The eyes should be protected with wraparound UVA-opaque glasses when exposed to sunlight directly or through window glass after ingestion of psoralen. The duration of this protection is a subject of some debate. The present guidelines for PUVA therapy suggest that UV-opaque glasses be worn from the time of exposure to psoralen until sunset on the day of treatment when patients are using sunlight for illumination. Earlier guidelines suggested eye protection for 24 or 48 hr. Patient compliance is an important consideration, and every effort must be made to ensure that suitable glasses are used during the most critical period, namely, the remainder of the day after ingestion of psoralen when exposed to sunlight. Skin sensitivity persists for up to 12 hr. Therefore, following ingestion of psoralen, the patient must avoid exposure to UVA radiation for the remainder of the day. Adequate clothing and avoidance of sunlight are the best protection. Sunscreens containing benzophenones and avobenzone partially protect against psoralen phototoxicity, as they have some absorption in the UVA waveband. Skin protection is most important after the first few treatments and in fair-skinned individuals.

Nontreatment Days

The patient is receiving a phototoxic treatment, and since risks are probably dose related, it is advisable to reduce all phototoxic insults to a minimum. Environmental exposure to UV radiation should be minimized by restricting deliberate sun exposure, regularly using a broad-spectrum sunscreen, and wearing UV-opaque sunglasses. As a result of PUVA therapy, most patients are pigmented, and this often encourages them to engage in greatly increased exposure to sunlight. For fair-skinned individuals, this is probably a very unwise attitude. In addition, a sunlight-induced tan complicates and probably reduces the effectiveness of treatment.

EDUCATION OF PATIENTS

There are three stages in the process of educating patients about the treatment (Table 13).

Initial Consultation

The physician begins the education process during the first consultation by explaining the nature of the treatment, the precautions that must be taken and the potential adverse effects. For example, it is wise to tell patients that there is a 10% chance of their developing a significant erythema during the clearance phase of treatment since a forewarned patient is more accepting of this adverse effect. Finally, the patient should be given a handout which

Table 13 Patient Education

Initial consultation
Nature of treatment
Potential adverse effects
Treatment handout
First treatment
Answer questions
Explain mechanics of treatment
Subsequent treatments
Time of ingestion of psoralen
Number of capsules taken
Use of eye protection
Avoidance of sunlight

---

explains the treatment and be invited to direct any questions that arise to the nurse at the time of the first treatment.

First Treatment

The nurse or technician performing the first treatment should have 10–15 min available to introduce the patient to the mechanics of the treatment. First, to check if the patient has taken methoxsalen, how many capsules, and at what time. Second, to check on the use of eye protection and avoidance of sunlight. Third, to explain how the treatment unit works and the safety features.

Subsequent Treatments

In addition to asking about the response to treatment and any problems that might have arisen, periodically during treatment patients should be questioned about the number and timing of the psoralen capsules they have taken, their use of eye protection, and their avoidance of exposure to sunlight on the days of treatment.

SHORT-TERM SIDE EFFECTS

Every treatment has adverse effects and PUVA therapy is no exception. There are several points to keep in mind when evaluating any problem:

- The treatment is new and different for most patients, and this leads to much anxiety and, consequently, many minor complaints.
- Many complaints have no connection with the therapy. Just because the patients are on PUVA therapy does not mean they

cannot develop other disorders, so it is wise not to be too hasty in ascribing every complaint to the treatment.

- The real short-term problems (Table 14) are usually minor and can be easily overcome, so that less than 1% of patients cease treatment because of adverse effects.

It is very important for the physician and staff to have a positive attitude, to be confident in what they are doing, to provide an adequate explanation when problems arise, and to show active interest in overcoming difficulties.

Side Effects Due to Methoxsalen Alone

Gastrointestinal Disturbances

Anorexia, nausea, and, less commonly, vomiting are problems with methoxsalen. They appear to be due to a central mechanism triggered by high serum levels of the drug. Sequential measures to overcome these problems are:

- Taking methoxsalen with food that has a high fat content to slow down absorption.

Table 14 Short-Term Side Effects

Due to methoxsalen
Gastrointestinal effects
CNS symptoms
Bronchoconstriction
Toxic hepatitis
Drug fever
Exanthema
Phototoxicity
Erythema
Pruritus
Subacute phototoxicity
Photo-onycholysis
Koebner Phenomenon
Friction blisters
Phytophotodermatitis
Ankle edema
Nonphototoxic reactions
Cardiovascular stress
Hypertrichosis
Herpes simplex
New rash[a]

---

[a]See problem cases in Chapter 20.

- Scheduling treatments for late in the day since symptoms are always more marked in the morning.
- Reducing the dose by 10 mg, provided the patient is taking 30–40 mg. Never reduce the dose below 20 mg in an adult since all effect of the treatment may be lost due to the first-pass effect by the liver.
- Splitting the dose so that half the dose is taken 90 min before treatment and the other half is taken 1 hr before treatment.
- Using an antiemetic such as Tigan.

The first two measures solve the problem in 90% of those affected, the third measure solves it in most of the rest, while the last two measures are only required in about one patient in a thousand.

CNS Disturbances

Symptoms related to the nervous system are the most common side effect of PUVA therapy if patients are questioned, but, fortunately, few voluntarily complain of these problems. Presumably, they result from a direct effect of methoxsalen on the brain since they can precede exposure to UVA radiation and UVA radiation does not penetrate through the cranium. The symptoms include headache, dizziness, light-headedness, depression, hyperkineticism, insomnia, and a feeling of detachment from the environment. These symptoms seldom require any attention except agreement with the patient that they are due to the therapy. Occasionally the dose of methoxsalen has to be reduced to alleviate the symptoms and about once a year a patient is forced to stop treatment because of them.

Bronchoconstriction

Six cases of asthma have been reported with an onset several hours after ingestion of methoxsalen and lasting hours to days. Some of the patients have had a history of asthma and most have developed the reaction after considerable exposure to the therapy. The bronchoconstriction is a reaction to the drug and exposure to UVA radiation is not required to induce it. Therapy for asthma was successful in controlling one patient but the remainder ceased treatment.

Hepatic Toxicity

Concern has been expressed in the past about the hepatic effects of PUVA therapy. However, there are only two reports of apparent toxic hepatitis associated with the treatment. Liver function tests performed on 1600 patients over a 3-year period showed no significant alterations and no differences were found in liver biopsies taken before and after a year of PUVA therapy in two separate studies. In addition, PUVA therapy has been used in many patients with liver failure without apparent deterioration.

Drug Fever

Three cases of a febrile reaction developing several hours after PUVA therapy have been reported. Presumably, this is an allergic hypersensitivity to the drug.

Exanthema

Development of a widespread maculopapular eruption following exposure to methoxsalen has been reported in three patients.

Phototoxic Reactions

Erythema

Symptomatic erythema is the most troubling adverse effect of PUVA therapy and unfortunately, regardless of the care and caution of the therapist it cannot be avoided in all patients.

Frequency: In several large studies it has been found that around 10% of patients will develop a symptomatic erythema during the clearance phase of the treatment. A symptomatic erythema was defined in these studies as an erythema causing at least one missed treatment.

Cause: The suspected causes of a phototoxic erythema in one large retrospective study are listed in Table 15. The commonest cause is patients reaching their threshold of tolerance for the treatment. This is tied in with the uncontrolled variable in the treatment, namely, intestinal absorption of methoxsalen. There is considerable individual variation in absorption and high absorbers are more prone to an acute erythemal response. Treatment on consecutive days on a T.I.W. or B.I.W. schedule and treating in the presence of an existing mild erythema are other contributing factors. Interestingly, technical errors and photosensitizing medications were uncommon causes.

Management: If an erythema is localized, for example, affecting just the breasts or buttocks, the area can be covered and treatment continued. If the erythema is more generalized, treatment should be stopped until it has completely resolved. Once it is known that a patient has widespread erythema, they should be seen and evaluated and follow-up should be on a regular basis until all symptoms subside.

There is no specific treatment for PUVA-induced erythema. Corticosteroids and prostaglandin synthetase inhibitors such as indomethacin do not influence the course of the erythemal response. Supportive measures such as cool baths, liberal use of moisturizing creams, aspirin, and antipruritics offer some relief. In addition, it is well to make sure the patient knows that symptoms are likely to persist for a minimum of 7 to 10 days and may last 2 to 3 weeks, depending on the severity of the erythema.

Table 15 Suspected Causes of Symptomatic Erythema

	No. of patients	Percentage of patients
Treatment protocol		61
Dose UVA too high	18	
High-absorption methoxsalen	6	
Therapy on consecutive days	3	
Addition of UVB	2	
Time of treatment	2	
Patient variable		21
Medications	3	
Compliance	7	
Concurrent disease	1	
Technical error	2	4
Unknown	7	14

Pruritus

Mild pruritus is a very common complaint. The most common cause of pruritus is dryness of the skin and it responds to lubricants. PUVA therapy can cause a second type of pruritus, commonly called the "PUVA itch," which is a deep, burning sensation, often likened to a feeling of something crawling under the skin. This is a symptom of phototoxicity and, while it is associated with all symptomatic erythemas, it can often occur as the sole evidence of excessive treatment. The outer aspects of the arms, thighs, breasts, and buttocks are the common sites. The mechanism of this symptom is not clear but probably involves phototoxic injury to dermal nerve endings.

Intense pruritus from phototoxicity is an indication to stop treatment until it completely clears, which may take 2 to 3 weeks. Symptomatic treatment, as for an erythemal reaction, provides some relief but antipruritics are of little help. Very occasionally, a patient continues to have pruritus for months despite cessation of treatment, and phenytoin in a dose of 150 mg B.I.D. and gabapentin up to 1200 mg per day have been reported to be useful in providing symptomatic relief. Consultation with a neurologist can also be useful in this difficult situation.

Subacute Phototoxicity

This syndrome consists of the sudden onset of a widespread psoriasiform eruption. It is an uncommon problem but important to diagnose since continuing treatment makes for a very uncomfortable patient. The patient usually believes they have had a sudden exacerbation of their psoriasis and wants an increase in treatment. The clue that this is not psoriasis is the intense pruritus which is always present, and then on physical examination the finding that all relatively unexposed areas; such as the inner thighs and axillae, are spared (Table 16). If in doubt, do a bilateral comparison (Chapter 5) covering one side and the answer will be apparent after a couple of treatments. A biopsy is not helpful since the pathology is psoriasiform hyperplasia.

Management of this condition is to stop treatment, oatmeal baths, moisturizers, and antipruritics and the eruption clears in 3 to 4 weeks. PUVA therapy cannot be resumed immediately because subacute phototoxicity will return even at lower doses. However, if an alternative treatment is used for 6–12 months, PUVA therapy at up to 50% of the original dose of UVA radiation is tolerated.

Photo-onycholysis

A few patients develop a painful, white or yellow discoloration of one or more nails during therapy, and this is a sign of phototoxicity in the nail bed. Application of an opaque nail polish prior to each treatment permits continuation of therapy with recovery of the nail. Interestingly, this adverse effect is most common in patients with vitiligo of the digits and is presumably due in part to a lack of melanocytes in the nail bed.

Pigmentation of the nail, melanonychia, is sometimes seen in dark-skinned patients as either distal even pigmentation or bands across the nails. This is asymptomatic and reversible once treatment is stopped.

Koebner Phenomenon

Patients with active, aggressive psoriasis are candidates for developing a Koebner response if their skin is injured by therapy. An erythemal reaction in normal skin or subacute phototoxicity must be carefully monitored to ensure that the appearance of this problem is not missed. A phototoxic reaction can be quickly superseded by psoriasis, and this is an indication to continue PUVA therapy at a level that will treat the disease but avoid

Table 16 Subacute Phototoxicity

The patient
Skin type I or II
Refractory psoriasis
The onset
Usually after more than 100 treatments
While on a clearance schedule
Preceding 1–2 weeks of pruritus, tingling or tightness of skin
Rash appears over 2–3 days
The appearance
Widespread psoriasiform eruption
Spares relatively nonexposed areas such as axillae and inner thighs

---

phototoxicity. Polymorphous light eruption is another event that can trigger a Koebner response, and PUVA therapy should never be stopped because of the appearance of this reaction.

Friction Blisters

A fairly common occurrence, particularly in patients being treated close to their erythema threshold, is the development of bullae on otherwise normal skin in association with friction or low-grade trauma. The sides of the hands and feet are the most common sites and new, tight-fitting shoes are a common trigger. Manual occupations, such as plumbing or carpentry, are other causes. PUVA therapy decreases adhesion at the dermoepidermal junction as evidenced by diminished time for suction blister formation, and this is probably the main factor in the formation of these bullae.

Phytophotodermatitis

Bizarre patterns of erythema, with or without associated blisters, followed by intense pigmentation suggests the diagnosis of phytophotodermatitis. Of course, this is a contradiction in terms to some extent since both phyto-photodermatitis and PUVA therapy involve an interaction of psoralen and UVA radiation. But there is a difference. Oral psoralens rarely if ever give rise to bullae. Recently, we observed this phytophotodermatitis reaction as a result of patients handling psoralen solution that had leaked from capsules; such accidental exposure to psoralens is probably the mechanism of all such reactions.

Ankle Edema

A few patients develop edema of the ankles as the first sign of phototoxicity. Usually there are other predisposing factors such as varicose veins or cardiac insufficiency. Sometimes the edema is unilateral. In either case it is essential to suspend treatment to investigate an underlying cause, and usually to reduce the dose of therapy.

Nonphotoxic Reactions

Cardiovascular Stress

There has been much discussion about the stress PUVA therapy exerts on the cardiovascular system, with agreement that the treatment causes some tachycardia. Anxiety associated with a new treatment and a high temperature in the radiator are probably the main causes of this change. A temperature of 40°C is typical in a radiator that is not air-conditioned. More serious problems such as arrhythmias have not been reported. Cardiovascular stress can be minimized by using short treatments and having adequate air-conditioning. A recent myocardial infarction and an unstable cardiac state are relative contraindications to treatment.

Hypertrichosis

This is very common in both men and women, but it is usually only remarked on by women. The most common complaint is increased prominence of facial hair that has become longer and darker. One study found that all patients treated with PUVA therapy had an increase in hair length. However, it is important to note that hirsuitism, or androgen-mediated growth of hair in women does not result from the treatment.

Herpes Simplex

The frequency of recurrent herpes labialis is increased in patients on PUVA therapy, but there is no evidence that primary infection is more common.

Other Cutaneous Disorders

These are discussed under Problem Cases (Chapter 20).

LONG-TERM SIDE EFFECTS

PUVA therapy has attracted more study of its long-term effects than any other treatment in dermatology and possibly in the whole of medicine. Large prospective studies were conducted in the United States and Europe and smaller studies have been conducted in other countries so that there are more than 25 years of follow-up data. To place this in context, the longest prospective study of a topical corticosteroid agent is about 12 weeks.

The study that has given us the most information is a 16-center prospective study of over 1300 patients (National Institutes of Health PUVA Follow-up Study; Robert Stern, Director) and these patients were started on therapy in 1975. It is important when evaluating the results from this study to keep a few points in focus. At the time the study was initiated PUVA therapy for psoriasis was experimental and was only available in those centers. Second, the only effective treatments available at the time for moderate-to-severe psoriasis were sunlight, the Goeckerman regimen, and methotrexate. Due to these limitations, each center entered their most severely affected patients and by definition these patients tended to have the most prior exposure to other treatments including other carcinogens. Third, almost all the patients were fair-skinned Caucasians. Finally, the exposure doses used at that time were much higher than are generally used today. Thus, this is the perfect study to look for adverse effects since it had a highly susceptible population exposed to high doses of treatment. The results from the study warn us about the adverse effect we are likely to see but the magnitude of the risk is probably exaggerated as compared to usual clinical practice.

Photoaging of the Skin

PUVA therapy produces changes in the skin that resemble photoaging induced by sunlight. Early in the course of therapy, the skin becomes dry and wrinkled; these changes are fully reversible on cessation of therapy. However, with long-term treatment the changes become more marked, with the appearance of telangiectasia and disturbance of melanization in the form of freckles and macules of hypopigmentation. These changes are only partially reversible. Photoaging is strongly related to skin type: patients with skin types I and II show the most marked changes, while little or no change is seen in skin types V and VI. Dose is also important, photoaging is more likely to occur and will be more marked with high exposure. The freckles seen in PUVA patients are really lentigines with an increase in the number of melanocytes. The average size of melanocytes is also increased and some cellular atypia can be seen in the so-called "PUVA lentigo," which can appear quite dark. There is no evidence that these lesions are precursors of melanoma.

Nonmelanoma Skin Cancer

Squamous Cell Carcinoma

Treatment with PUVA therapy is clearly associated with an increased risk of developing squamous cell carcinoma (SCC) and in fair-skinned Caucasians about 10% of patients will develop these tumors if they receive high doses of therapy. The factors that increase the risk are listed in Table 17. These factors are both cumulative and independent in their effects. For example, a person with skin type III probably reaches a threshold of risk for SCC beyond 250 treatments while a patient with a past history of skin cancer or with actinic keratoses has reached the threshold at the start of treatment. Many of these tumors occur on non-sun-exposed skin, the tumors are frequently multiple, and metastases have occurred in up to 5% of patients, particularly in males with tumors on the genitalia. The cause and effect relationship is strongly supported by a strong dose–response relationship. There is some evidence that oral retinoids reduce the risk of developing SCC.

Table 17 Factors Increasing Risk of SCC

Low skin types I–III
High dose of PUVA (>250 Tx)
P/H skin cancer
Presence of actinic keratoses
Treatment with cyclosporine

Basal Cell Carcinoma

A small but significantly increased risk of basal cell carcinoma (BCC) has been observed in the multicenter study in the United States with lesions mainly occurring on the trunk. Other studies have not confirmed this finding.

Keratoacanthomas

This tumor is reported to be more common in some studies.

Merkel Cell Carcinoma

Three cases of this rare tumor have been reported in PUVA-treated patients and these patients had a history of BCC and SCC.

Melanoma

An increased incidence of melanoma began to appear in the multicenter study 15 years after the start of treatment and the incidence has increased steadily. This has not been observed in other studies but the duration and completeness of follow-up in those studies may be inadequate. It should be noted that SCC remains the primary cause of cancer morbidity and mortality in psoriasis patients treated with PUVA therapy. The risk of developing melanoma is about the same as the risk of developing metastatic SCC.

Ocular Changes

The potential ocular risk of PUVA therapy is cataracts. In evaluating the risk of cataractogenesis from PUVA therapy, there are several pieces of information to be considered:

- PUVA treatment in high doses causes cataracts in mice and rats. In lower doses, closer to those used in humans, PUVA treatment did not cause cataracts in rabbits during 18 months of exposure. These findings probably indicate a difference in susceptibility between species and possibly an effect of dose.
- Methoxsalen does enter the lens in humans and exposure to UVA radiation induces the formation of photoproducts. It is not known how long free methoxsalen remains in the lens, but in animals it can be detected 12 hr after administration.
- There are anecdotal reports of several patients who developed cataracts following a course of PUVA therapy and who did not use adequate eye protection.
- Large prospective studies of patients receiving PUVA therapy over 5–10 years have not revealed an increased frequency of cataracts.

- The frequency of cataracts in patients with psoriasis appears to be similar to that in the normal population.

Systemic Neoplasia

There have been suggestions from several studies of various systemic malignancies being associated with PUVA therapy but there is no consistency in these reports.

Immunosuppression

PUVA therapy is clearly immunosuppressive in both animal and human studies but there is no evidence that this has clinical relevance.

Hepatic Toxicity

Concern has been expressed in the past about the hepatic effect of PUVA therapy, and since its widespread use, there have been several case reports of hepatitis associated with the treatment. However, if this association is true, it is almost certainly an idiosyncratic effect. Liver function tests performed on 1500 patients over a 3-year period showed no significant alteration, and no significant differences were found in liver biopsy samples taken before and after 1 year of PUVA treatment in 35 patients. In addition, PUVA therapy has been used in patients with liver failure without any apparent deterioration.

GUIDELINES FOR USE OF PUVA THERAPY

PUVA therapy is carcinogenic producing an increased risk of developing SCC and possibly also melanoma. Therefore, certain guidelines should be considered in its use.

General Considerations

- Skin cancer is mainly a risk in skin types I–III and in the absence of other risk factors is probably not a risk in skin types IV–VI. Skin cancer is less of a risk in older patients due to the latency period for development of tumors.
- An aim of treatment should be to keep the exposure dose as low as possible in terms of total dose of UVA radiation and number of treatments.

Approach to Therapy

- There are a number of treatments available for moderate-to-severe psoriasis and also for certain other diseases treated with PUVA

therapy and these should be considered when developing a treatment plan. However, these treatments may also have potential long-term risks.
- Combination therapy for the clearance phase of treatment and rotational therapy may be used to reduce the overall exposure to PUVA therapy.

Monitoring of Patients

- Early detection of skin cancer is key to successful treatment and patients require teaching about self-examination and physicians need to maintain an open-door policy for examination of suspect lesions.
- Protection of the genitalia in men and the face in everyone, if these areas are not affected by disease, reduces the risks of treatment.

OTHER FORMS OF ORAL PUVA THERAPY

PUVAsol Therapy

The sun is a very effective source of UVA radiation and also has the additional advantage of being free. However, it does have some disadvantages including variations in the UVA irradiance during the course of the day plus wide seasonal variation, variability and unpredictability of the weather, a high content of UVB radiation, and the difficulty of finding a private, insect-free location for whole-body exposure.

PUVAsol therapy with oral methoxsalen is effective in clearing psoriasis. However, in a study of the efficacy of this treatment in a clinic setting, one-third of patients had symptomatic erythema, which is far higher than with artificial sources of radiation. This occurred despite the use of an integrating spectroradiometer to ensure that each patient received the correct dose of UVA radiation. Presumably, a narrow margin between the therapeutic and phototoxic doses of the therapy is responsible for this problem. The message from these observations is that if the sun is to be used as a source of UVA radiation with methoxsalen as the photosensitizer, accurate radiometry is essential to overcome the problem of varying irradiance with time and cloud cover; purchase of this expensive equipment will be of little interest to most therapists.

Do-It-Yourself PUVA Therapy

Frequent visits to a treatment center or a physician's office are a nuisance for most patients, and this occasionally leads to suggestions for Do-It-Yourself (DIY) PUVA therapy at home or elsewhere. Several sources of UVA radiation have been used in combination with methoxsalen, and while none of these is safe, the reason for the lack of safety varies with the circumstances.

- Sun is a favored source of radiation because it is cheap and the hazards of PUVAsol therapy have already been mentioned.
- Many suntan parlors now use UVA lamps, and they have been advocated by a few as a way of conducting DIY therapy. The emission spectra of UVA lamps in suntan parlors are very variable and unknown to both the proprietor and any physician who considers their use. Thus, the spectrum might be more or less effective in activating methoxsalen, and therefore the patient might not clear or might be severely burned.
- Purchase of a PUVA radiator is contemplated by some patients, and, apart from the expense and lack of control of therapy, this has all the disadvantages of home UVB phototherapy. Besides, most manufacturers of this equipment will not sell directly to patients.
- UVB sunlamp bulbs have been used in combination with methoxsalen but, as already mentioned, the emission spectrum of these lamps is not effective in activating psoralen, and UVB-induced phototoxicity occurs before any phototherapeutic benefit of the UVA/psoralen reaction.

DIY PUVA therapy with methoxsalen has all the hallmarks of an uncontrolled hit-or-miss treatment and has nothing to recommend it for either the patient or the physician; it should only be embarked on by therapists who are very well insured.

Oral 5-Methoxypsoralen Photochemotherapy

Bergapten, or 5-methoxypsoralen, has been used in Europe for about 10 years in the therapy of psoriasis. Originally, the compound was used in a microcrystalline form, but it is now available as a solution in a soft gelatin capsule and this formulation gives better absorption. However, the serum levels obtained with 5-methoxypsoralen are only about 25% of those with methoxsalen when equal doses are given. Thus, the current recommendation is to use 1.2 mg/kg body weight of 5-methoxypsoralen, which gives half the serum level obtained with 0.6 mg/kg body weight of methoxsalen. Despite this difference, in a between-patient, comparison study, patients treated with 5-methoxypsoralen had almost as good a response to treatment as patients treated with methoxsalen, when the doses were 1.2 vs. 0.6 mg, respectively.

5-Methoxypsoralen in these studies has had some advantages over methoxsalen. It does not appear to cause nausea or other gastrointestinal disturbances and is less prone to cause erythema and pruritus. Of course, this better profile of short-term side effects may just be a reflection of poorer absorption and lower serum levels, and it remains to be proven in larger studies that therapeutic efficacy is not being sacrificed. A transient maculo-papular eruption on relatively nonexposed areas was observed in some patients during treatment with 5-methoxypsoralen and UVA radiation; the pathogenesis of this phenomenon is unexplained.

Oral Trisoralen Photochemotherapy

A few investigators have advocated the use of trimethylpsoralen in treat-ment, but, in general, experience has been disappointing. Trisoralen is poorly absorbed after oral administration and much less phototoxic than methoxsalen when the same dose of the two agents is ingested. We have had an occasional patient with both vitiligo and psoriasis report that psor-iasis responds to trisoralen and sunlight, but this combination has not been studied; the response may have been due to solar UVB radiation.

BIBLIOGRAPHY

Guidelines

Drake LA, Ceilley RI, Dorner W, Goltz RW, Graham GF, Lewis CW, Salasche SJ, Turner MLC, Lowery BJ. Guidelines of care for photo-therapy and photochemotherapy. J Am Acad Dermatol 1994; 31:643–648.
British Photodermatology Group. British Photodermatology Group guide-lines for PUVA. Br J Dermatol 1994; 130:246–255.

Methoxsalen

Brickl R, Schmid J, Koss FW. Clinical pharmacology of oral psoralen drugs. Photodermatology 1984; 174–186.
Hönigsmann H, Jaschke EJ, Nitsche V, Brenner W, Rauschmeier W, Wolff K. Serum levels of 8-methoxypsoralen in two different drug prepara-tions: correlation with photosensitivity and UV-A dose requirements for photochemotherapy. J Invest Dermatol 1982; 79:233–236.
Jansen CT, Wilen G, Paul R. Variations in skin photosensitization during repeated oral 8-methoxypsoralen medication. Arch Dermatol Res 1983; 275:315–317.
Levins PC, Gange RW, Momtaz TK, Parrish JA, Fitzpatrick TB. A new liquid formulation of 8-methoxypsoralen: bioactivity and effect of diet. J Invest Dermatol 1984; 82:185–187.
Lowe NJ, Urbach F, Bailin P, Weingarten DP. Comparative efficacy of two dosage forms of oral methoxsalen in psoralens plus ultraviolet A ther-apy of psoriasis. J Am Acad Dermatol 1987; 16:994–998.

Sullivan TJ, Walter JL, Kouba RF, et al. Bioavailability of a new oral methoxsalen formulation. Arch Dermatol 1986; 122:768–771.

Van Boven M, Roelandts R, DeGreef H, Kinget R, Adriaens P, Daenens P. A pharmacokinetic comparison in dogs of seven brands of 8-MOP and five new formulations. Photodermatology 1985; 2:27–31.

UVA Radiation

Carabott FM, Hawk JLM. A modified dosage schedule for increased efficiency in PUVA treatment of psoriasis. Clin Exp Dermatol 1989; 14:337–340.

Jansen CT. Self-reported skin type and reactivity to UVB, UVA and PUVA irradiation. Photodermatology 1989; 6:234–236.

Rampen FHJ, Fleuren BAM, DeBoo TM, Lemmens WAJG. Unreliability of self-reported burning tendency and tanning ability. Arch Dermatol 1988; 124:885–888.

Stern RS, Momtaz TK. Skin typing for assessment of skin cancer risk and acute response to UV-B and oral methoxsalen photochemotherapy. Arch Dermatol 1984; 120:869–873.

Wolff K, Gschnait F, Hönigsmann H, Konrad K, Parrish JA, Fitzpatrick TB. Phototesting and dosimetry for photochemotherapy. Br J Dermatol 1977; 96:1–10.

Schedules for Clearing Psoriasis

Buckley DA, Phillips WG. 8-methoxypsoralen PUVA for psoriasis: a comparison of a minimal phototoxic dose-based regimen with a skin-type approach. Br J Dermatol 1997; 136:800–801.

Collins P, Wainwright NJ, Amorim I, Lakshmipathi T, Ferguson J. 8-MOP PUVA for psoriasis: a comparison of a minimal phototoxic dose-based regimen with a skin-type approach. Br J Dermatol 1996; 135:248–254.

Diette KM, Momtaz TK, Stern RS, Arndt KA, Parrish JA. Psoralens and UV-A and UV-B twice weekly for the treatment of psoriasis. Arch Dermatol 1984; 120:1169–1173.

Gupta AK, Anderson TF. Psoralen photochemotherapy. J Am Acad Dermatol 1987; 17:703–734.

Melski JW, Tanenbaum L, Parrish JA, Fitzpatrick TB, Bleich HL, and 28 participating investigators. Oral methoxsalen photochemotherapy for the treatment of psoriasis: a cooperative clinical trial. J Invest Dermatol 1977; 68:328–335.

Momtaz TK, Parrish JA. Combination of psoralens and ultraviolet A and ultraviolet B in the treatment of psoriasis vulgaris: a bilateral comparison study. J Am Acad Dermatol 1984; 10:481–486.

Morison WL, Parrish JA, Fitzpatrick TB. Controlled study of PUVA and adjunctive topical therapy in the management of psoriasis. Br J Dermatol 1978; 98:125–132.

Parrish JA, Fitzpatrick TB, Tanenbaum L, Pathak MA. Photochemotherapy of psoriasis with oral methoxsalen and longwave ultraviolet light. N Engl J Med 1974; 291:1207–1211.

Roenigk HH and 19 participating investigators. Photochemotherapy for psoriasis. Arch Dermatol 1979; 115:576–579.

Wolff K, Fitzpatrick TB, Parrish JA, Gschnait P, Gilchrest B, Hönigsmann H, Pathak MA, Tannanbaum L. Photochemotherapy for psoriasis with orally administered methoxsalen. Arch Dermatol 1986; 112:943–950.

Response to PUVA Therapy

Marx JL, Scher RK. Response of psoriatic nails to oral photochemotherapy. Arch Dermatol 1980; 116:1023–1024.

Perlman SG, Gerber LH, Roberts M, Nigra TP, Barth WF. Photochemotherapy and psoriatic arthritis. Ann Intern Med 1979; 91:717–722.

Maintenance Therapy

Melski JW, Stern RS. Annual rate of psoralen and ultraviolet-A treatment of psoriasis after initial clearing. Arch Dermatol 1982; 118:404–408.

Stern RS. Long-term use of psoralens and ultraviolet A for psoriasis: evidence for efficacy and cost savings. J Am Acad Dermatol 1986; 14: 520–526.

Stern RS, Melski JW. Long-term continuation of psoralen and ultraviolet A treatment of psoriasis. Arch Dermatol 1982; 118:400–403.

Short-Term Problems

Anderson CD, Frondin T. Unusual adverse effects of 8-methoxypsoralen: bronchial reaction during photochemotherapy (PUVA). J Am Acad Dermatol 1984; 10:298.

Baran R, Juhlin L. Drug-induced photo-onycholysis. J Am Acad Dermatol 1978; 17:1012–1016.

Berg M. Drug fever caused by 8-methoxypsoralen. Photodermatology 1989; 6:149–150.

Bjellerup B, Bruze M, Hansson A, Krook G, Ljunggren B. Liver injury following administration of 8-methoxypsoralen during PUVA therapy. Acta Dermatol 1979; 59:371–372.

Chappe SG, Roenigk HH, Miller AJ, Beeaff DE, Tyrpin L. The effect of photochemotherapy on the cardiovascular system. J Am Acad Dermatol 1981; 4:561–565.

Ciafone RA, Rhodes AR, Audley M, Freedberg IM, Abelmann WH. The cardiovascular stress of photochemotherapy (PUVA). J Am Acad Dermatol 1980; 3:499–505.

Cox NH, Rogers S. Cutaneous drug eruption caused by 8-methoxypsoralen. Photodermatology 1989; 6:96–97.

Friedman PS, Coburn P, Dahl MGC, Diffey BL, Ross J, Ford GP, Parker SC, Bird P. PUVA-induced blisters, complement deposition, and damage to the dermoepidermal junction. Arch Dermatol 1987; 123: 1471–1477.

Gisslen P, Kalimo K, Larko O. Exanthematous drug reaction caused by 8-methoxypsoralen. Photodermatology 1986; 3:308–309.

Hann SK, Kwang SY, Park Y. Melanonychia induced by systemic photochemotherapy. Photodermatology 1989; 6:98–99.

Jordon WP. PUVA, pruritus, and the loss of the axon flare. Arch Dermatol 1978; 115:636.

Kasa IT, Dobozy A. Drug fever caused by PUVA treatment. Acta Dermatol Venereol (Stockh) 1985; 65:557–558.

Kumakiri M, Hasimoto K. Cutaneous nerve stimulation by psoralen-ultraviolet A therapy: an ultrastructural study. J Invest Dermatol 1978; 70:163–172.

Kumakiri M, Hashimoto K, Willis I. Biological changes of human cutaneous nerves caused by ultraviolet irradiation: an ultrastructural study. Br J Dermatol 1978; 99:65–72.

Mackie RM. Onycholysis occurring during PUVA therapy. Clin Exp Dermatol 1979; 4:111–112.

Morison WL. Topical phototoxicity from oral methoxsalen capsules. Arch Dermatol 1989; 125:433–434.

Morison WL, Marwaha S, Beck L. PUVA-induced phototoxicity: incidence and causes. J Am Acad Dermatol 1997; 36:183–185.

Morison WL. Subacute phototoxicity caused by treatment with oral psoralen plus UV-A. Arch Dermatol 1997; 133:1609.

Naik RPC, Parameswara YR. 8-Methoxypsoralen-induced nail pigmentation. Int J Dermatol 1982; 21:275–277.

Norris PG, Maurice PDL, Schott GD, Greaves MW. Persistent skin pain after PUVA. Clin Exp Dermatol 1987; 12:403–405.

Pariser DM, Wyles RJ. Toxic hepatitis from oral methoxsalen photochemotherapy (PUVA). J Am Acad Dermatol 1980; 3:248–250.

Prens EP, Smeenk G. Effect of photochemotherapy on the cardiovascular system. Dermatologica 1983; 167:208–211.

Rampen RHJ. Hypertrichosis in PUVA-treated patients. Br J Dermatol 1983; 109:657–660.

Rampen FHJ, Hypertrichosis: a side-effect of PUVA therapy. Arch Dermatol Res 1985; 278:82–83.

Ramsay B, Marks JM. Bronchoconstriction due to 8-methoxypsoralen. Br J Dermatol 1988; 119:83–86.

Rau RC, Flowers FP, Barrett JL. Photo-onycholysis secondary to psoralen use. Arch Dermatol 1978; 14:448.

Ravenscroft J, Goulden V, Wilkinson M. Systemic allergic contact dermatitis to 8-methoxypsoralen (8-MOP). J Am Acad Dermatol 2001; 45:S218–S219.

Roelandts R, Lonche J, Degreff H. Phytophotodermatitis-like lesion induced by PUVA. Photodermatology 1985; 2:40–43.

Weiss E, Sayegh-Carreno R. PUVA-induced pigmented nails. Int J Dermatol 1989; 28:188–189.

Wennerstein G. Exacerbation of bronchial asthma during photochemotherapy with 8-methoxypsoralen and UVA (PUVA). Photodermatology 1987; 4:212–213.

Zala L, Omar A, Krebs A. Photo-onycholysis-induced by 8-methoxypsoralen. Dermatologica 1977; 154:203–215.

Zamiri M, Bilsland D. Treatment of bath PUVA-induced skin pain with gabapentin. Br J Dermatol 2004; 150:516–517.

Premature Aging

Green I, Cox AJ. Amyloid deposition after psoriasis therapy with psoralen and long-wave ultraviolet light. Arch Dermatol 1979; 115:1200–1202.

Gschnait F, Wolff K, Hönigsmann H, Stingl G, Brenner W, Jaschke E, Konrad K. Long-term photochemotherapy: histopathological and immunofluorescence observations in 243 patients. Br J Dermatol 1980; 103:11–22.

Hashimoto K, Kumakiri M. Colloid-amyloid bodies in PUVA-treated human psoriatic patients. J Invest Dermatol 1979; 72:70–80.

Kanerva L, Lauharanta J, Niemi KM, Juvakoski T, Lassus A. Persistent ashen-gray maculae and freckles induced by long-term PUVA treatment. Dermatologica 1983; 166:281–286.

Kanerva L, Niemi KM, Lauharanta J. A semiquantitative light and electron microscopic analysis of histopathologic changes in photochemotherapy-induced freckles. Arch Dermatol Res 1984; 276:2–11.

Kietzmann H, Christophers E. Pigmentary lesions after PUVA treatment. Dermatologica 1984; 168:306–308.

Levin DL, Roenigk HH, Caro WA. Histologic, immunofluorescent, and anti-nuclear antibody findings in PUVA-treated patients. J Am Acad Dermatol 1982; 6:328–333.

Niemi KM, Niemi A, Kanerva L. Morphologic changes in epidermis of PUVA-treated patients with psoriasis with or without a history of arsenic therapy. Arch Dermatol 1983; 119:904–909.

Oikarinen A, Karvonen J, Uitto J, et al. Connective tissue alterations in skin exposed to natural and therapeutic UV-radiation. Photodermatology 1985; 2:15–26.

Rhodes AR, Harrist TJ, Momtaz TK. The PUVA-induced pigmented macule: a lentiginous proliferation of large, sometimes cytologically atypical, melanocytes. J Am Acad Dermatol 1983; 9:47–58.

Rhodes AR, Stern RS, Melski JW. The PUVA lentigo: an analysis of predisposing factors. J Invest Dermatol 1983; 81:459–463.

Schuler G, Hönigsmann H, Jaschke E, Wolff K. Selective accumulation of lipid within melanocytes during photochemotherapy (PUVA) of psoriasis. Br J Dermatol 1982; 107:173–182.

Stern RS, Parrish JA, Fitzpatrick TB. Actinic degeneration in association with long-term use of PUVA. J Invest Dermatol 1985; 84:135–138.

Stern RS. Actinic degeneration and pigmentary change in association with psoralen and UVA treatment: a 20-year prospective study. J Am Acad Dermatol 2003; 48:61–67.

Zelickson AS, Mottaz JH, Zelickson BD, Muller SA. Elastic tissue changes in skin following PUVA therapy. J Am Acad Dermatol 1980; 3:186–192.

Skin Cancer

Bruynzeel I, Bergman W, Hartevelt HM, Kenter CCA, van de Velde EA, Schothorst AA, Suurmond D. 'High single-dose' European PUVA regimen also causes an excess of non-melanoma skin cancer. Br J Dermatol 1991; 124:49–55.

Eskelinen A, Halme K, Lassus A, Idänpään-Heikkulä J. Risk of cutaneous carcinoma in psoriatic patients treated with PUVA. Photodermatology 1985; 2:10–14.

Gritiyarangsan P, Sindhavananda J, Rungrairatanaroj P, Kullavanijaya P. Cutaneous carcinoma and PUVA lentigines in Thai patients treated with oral PUVA. Photodermatol Photoimmunol Photomed 1995; 11: 174–177.

Hannuksela-Svahn A, Pukkala E, Läärä E, Poikolainen K, Karvonen J. Psoriasis, its treatment, and cancer in a cohort of Finnish patients. J Invest Dermatol 2000; 114:587–590.

Henseler T, Christophers E, Hönigsmann H, Wolff K, and 19 other investigators. Skin tumors in the European PUVA Study. J Am Acad Dermatol 1987; 16:108–116.

Hönigsmann H, Wolff K, Gchnait F. Keratoses and nonmelanoma skin tumors in long-term photochemotherapy (PUVA). J Am Acad Dermatol 1980; 3:406–414.

Lindelöf B, Sigurgeirsson B, Tegner E, Larkö O, Johannesson A, Berne B, Christensen OB, Andersson T, Törngren M, Molin L, Nylander

Lundqvist E, Emtestam L. PUVA and cancer: a large-scale epidemiological study. Lancet 1991; 338:91–93.

Lindskov R. Skin carcinomas and treatment with photochemotherapy (PUVA). Acta Dermatol Venereol (Stockh) 1983; 63:223–226.

Lobel E, Paver K, King R, Le Guay J, Poyzer K, Wargon O. The relationship of skin cancer to PUVA therapy in Australia. Aust J Dermatol 1981; 22:100–103.

Lunder EJ, Stern RS. Merkel-cell carcinomas in patients treated with methoxsalen and ultraviolet A radiation. New Engl J Med 1998; 339: 1247–1248.

Marcil I, Stern RS. Squamous-cell cancer of the skin in patients given PUVA and ciclosporin: nested cohort crossover study. Lancet 2001; 358:1042–1045.

Margolis D, Bilker W, Hennessy S, Vittorio C, Santanna J, Strom BL. The risk of malignancy associated with psoriasis. Arch Dermatol 2001; 137:778–783.

Morison WL, Baughman RD, Day RM, Forbes D, Hönigsmann H, Krueger GG, Lebwohl M, Lew R, Naldi L, Parrish JA, Piepkorn M, Stern RS, Weinstein GD, Whitmore E. Consensus workshop on the toxic effects of long-term PUVA therapy. Arch Dermatol 1998; 134:595–598.

Nijsten TEC, Stern RS. The increased risk of skin cancer is persistent after discontinuation of psoralen + ultraviolet A: a cohort study. J Invest Dermatol 2003; 121:252–258.

Nijsten TEC, Stern RS. Oral retinoid use reduces cutaneous squamous cell carcinoma risk in patients with psoriasis treated with psoralen-UVA: a nested cohort study. J Am Acad Dermatol 2003; 49:644–650.

Paul CF, Ho VC, McGeown C, Christophers E, Schmidtmann B, Guillaume JC, Lamarque V, Dubertret L. Risk of malignancies in psoriasis patients treated with cyclosporine: a 5 y cohort study. J Invest Dermatol 2003; 120:211–216.

Roenigk HH, Caro WA. Skin cancer in the PUVA-48 cooperative study. J Am Acad Dermatol 1981; 4:319–324.

Ros AM, Wennersten G, Lagerholm B. Long-term photochemotherapy for psoriasis: a histopathological and clinical follow-up study with special emphasis on tumor incidence and behavior of pigmented lesions. Acta Dermatol Venereol (Stockh) 1983; 63:215–221.

Seidl H, Kreimer-Erlacher H, Bäck B, Soyer HP, Höfler G, Kerl H, Wolf P. Ultraviolet exposure as the main initiator of p53 mutations in basal cell carcinomas from psoralen and ultraviolet-A treated patients with psoriasis. J Invest Dermatol 2001; 117:365–370.

Stern RS, Laird N, Melski J, et al. Cutaneous squamous-cell carcinoma in patients treated with PUVA. N Engl J Med 1984; 310:1156–1161.

Stern RS, Nichols KT, Väkevä LH. Malignant melanoma in patients treated for psoriasis with methoxsalen (psoralen) and ultraviolet A radiation (PUVA). N Engl J Med 1997; 336:1041–1045.

Stern RS, Lange R. Non-melanoma skin cancer occurring in patients treated with PUVA five to ten years after first treatment. J Invest Dermatol 1988; 91:120–124.

Stern RS, Bagheri S, Nichols K. The persistent risk of genital tumors among men treated with psoralen plus ultraviolet A (PUVA) for psoriasis. J Am Acad Dermatol 2002; 47:33–39.

Stern RS, Thibodeau LA, Kleinerman RA, Parrish JA, Fitzpatrick TB, and 22 participating investigators. Risk of cutaneous carcinoma in patients treated with oral methoxsalen photochemotherapy for psoriasis. N Engl J Med 1979; 300:809–813.

Stern RS, Lunder EJ. Risk of squamous cell carcinoma and methoxsalen (psoralen) and UV-A radiation (PUVA). Arch Dermatol 1998; 134:1582–1585.

Tanew A, Hönigsmann H, Ortel B. Non melanoma skin tumors in long-term photochemotherapy treatment of psoriasis. J Am Acad Dermatol 1986; 15:960–965.

Torinuki W, Tagami H. Incidence of skin cancer in Japanese psoriatic patients treated with either methoxsalen phototherapy, Goeckerman regimen, or both therapies. J Am Acad Dermatol 1988; 18:1278–1281.

The Eye

Abdullah AN, Keczkes K. Cutaneous and ocular side-effects of PUVA photochemotherapy—a 10-year follow-up study. Clin Exp Dermatol 1989; 14:421–424.

Boukes RJ, Bruynzeel DP. Ocular findings in 340 long-term treated PUVA patients. Photodermatology 1985; 2:178–180.

Cloud TM, Hakim R, Griffin C. Photosensitization of the eye with methoxsalen. Arch Opthalmol 1961; 66:689–694.

Cyrlin MN, Pedvis-Leftick A, Sugar J. Cataract formation in association with ultraviolet photosensitivity. Arch Opthalmol 1980; 12:786–790.

Lerman S, Megaw J, Willis I. Potential ocular complications from PUVA therapy and their prevention. J Invest Dermatol 1980; 74:197–199.

Marqversen J, Axelsen I, Nielsen E, Zachariae H. 8-Methoxypsoralen and the eye. Arch Dermatol Res 1981; 270:387–390.

Parrish JA, Anderson RR, Urbach F. Effects of ultraviolet radiation on the eye. In: Biological Effects of Ultraviolet Radiation with Emphasis on Human Responses to Longwave Ultraviolet. New York: Plenum Press, 1978:177–220.

Parrish JA, Chylack LT, Woehler ME, Cheng HM, Pathak MA, Morison WL, Krugler J, Nelson WF. Dermatological and ocular examination in rabbits chronically photosensitized with methoxsalen. J Invest Dermatol 1979; 73:256–258.

Pedvis-Leftick A, Cyrlin MN, Solomon LM. Cataracts in a patient with vitiligo who received photochemotherapy. Arch Dermatol 1979; 115: 1253–1255.

Prystowsky JH, Keen MS, Rabinowitz AD, Stevens AW, DeLeo VA. Present status of eyelid phototherapy. J Am Acad Dermatol 1992; 26: 607–613.

Ronnerfalt L, Lydahl E, Wennersten G, et al. Opthalmological study of patients undergoing long-term PUVA therapy. Acta Derma Venereol (Stockh) 1982; 62:501–505.

Stern RS and the Photochemotherapy Follow-up Study. Ocular findings in patients treated with PUVA. J Invest Dermatol 1994; 103:534–538.

Taylor HR, West SK, Rosenthal FS, Muñoz B, Newland HS, Abbey H, Emmet EA. Effect of ultraviolet radiation on cataract formation. N Engl J Med 1988; 319:1429–1433.

Wanscher B, Vesterdal E. Syndermatotic cataract in patients with psoriasis. Acta Dermatol Venereol (Stockh) 1976; 56:397–399.

Woo TY, Wong RC, Wong JM, Wong JM, Anderson TF, Lerman S. Lenticular psoralen photoproducts and cataracts of a PUVA-treated psoriatic patient. Arch Dermatol 1985; 121:1307.

Immunity

Morison WL. Effects of ultraviolet radiation on the immune system in humans. Photochem Photobiol 1989; 50:515–524.

Morison WL, Kripke ML. Photoimmunology and skin cancer. Photochem Photobiol 1987; suppl:467–474.

Systemic Neoplasia

Freeman K, Warin AP. Acute myelomonocytic leukaemia developing in a patient with psoriasis treated with oral 8-methoxypsoralen and long-wave ultraviolet light. Clin Exp Dermatol 1985; 10:144–146.

Hansen NE. Development of acute myeloid leukaemia in a patient with psoriasis treated with oral 8-methoxypsoralen and longwave ultraviolet light. Scand J Haematol 1979; 22:57–60.

Sheehan-Dare RA, Cotterill JA, Barnard DL. Transformation of myelodysplasia to acute myeloid leukaemia during psoralen photochemotherapy (PUVA) treatment of psoriasis. Acta Dermatol Venereol (Stockh) 1988; 69:262–264.

Stern RS, Lange R. Cardiovascular disease, cancer, and cause of death in patients with psoriasis: 10 years prospective experience in a cohort of 1,380 patients. J Invest Dermatol 1988; 91:197–201.

Wagner J, Manthorpe R, Philip P. Preleukaemia (haemopoietic dysplasia) developing in a patient with psoriasis treated with 8-methoxypsoralen and ultraviolet light (PUVA treatment). Scand J Haematol 1978; 21:299–304.

Hepatic Function

Bjelerup M, Bruze M, Hansson A, et al. Liver injury following administration of 8-methoxypsoralen during PUVA therapy. Acta Dermatol Venereol (Stockh) 1979; 59:371.

Nyfors A, Dahl-Nyfors B, Hopwood D. Liver biopsies from patients with psoriasis related to photochemotherapy (PUVA): findings before and after 1 year of therapy in twelve patients. J Am Acad Dermatol 1986; 14:43–48.

Pariser DM, Wyles RJ. Toxic hepatitis from oral methoxsalen photochemotherapy. J Am Acad Dermatol 1980; 3:248–250.

Zachariae H, Kragballe K, Sogaard H. Liver biopsy in PUVA-treated patients. Acta Dermatol Venereol (Stockh) 1978; 59:268–270.

Other Forms of Oral PUVA Therapy

Becker SW. Trisoralen photochemotherapy. Aust J Dermatol 1977; 18: 15–19.

Hönigsmann H, Jaschke E, Gschnait F, Brenner W, Fritsch P, Wolff K. 5-Methoxypsoralen (Bergapten) in photochemotherapy of psoriasis. Br J Dermatol 1979; 101:369–378.

Parrish JA, White AD, Kingsbury T, Zahar M, Fitzpatrick TB. Photochemotherapy of psoriasis using methoxsalen and sunlight. Arch Dermatol 1977; 113:1529–1532.

Tanew A, Ortel B, Rappersberger K, Hönigsmann H. 5-Methoxypsoralen (Bergapten) for photochemotherapy. J Am Acad Dermatol 1988; 18:333–338.

Wamer W, Giles A, Kornhauser A. Kinetics of 8-methoxypsoralen and 5-methoxypsoralen distribution in guinea pig serum, epidermis and ocular lens. Photodermatology 1987; 4:236–239.

10

Topical PUVA Therapy

INTRODUCTION

Direct application of psoralen to the skin combined with subsequent exposure to UVA radiation has been used for treatment of psoriasis for almost as long as oral PUVA. The first approach used a dilute solution of trimethylpsoralen in a bath and subsequent studies have used methoxsalen and 5-methoxypsoralen in bath solutions as well as creams, gels, and lotions. Topical PUVA therapy is used most widely in Europe and it appears to be much less popular elsewhere. Since methoxsalen is the only psoralen available for use in the United States, the first part of this chapter will only discuss treatment with this agent, and other psoralens will be discussed separately.

PHARMACOLOGY

Absorption of Psoralen

The kinetics of psoralen absorption and photosensitivity after topical application depend on several variables. When using a dilute solution of methoxsalen as in bath or soak PUVA therapy the main determinants of photosensitivity are those listed in Table 1.

Concentration of the Solution

An increase of the concentration of the solution from 0.5 to 5 mg/L decreases the MPD by about 60%.

Table 1 Factors Influencing Photosensitivity from Exposure to a Dilute Methoxsalen Solution

Concentration of solution
Duration of immersion
Water temperature
Intra- and interindividual variation
Number of exposures
Body site
Presence of disease

Duration of Immersion

Increasing immersion time from 5 to 30 min reduces the MPD by about 60%.

Water Temperature

Increase in water temperature has a small effect on photosensitivity with the lowest MPD around 37°C.

Intraindividual and Interindividual Variation

Small variations of the MPD are observed on repeated testing of the same individuals and a much larger variation is seen in different people. In addition, there is a poor correlation between skin types II and III and the MPD.

Number of Exposures

Five treatments over the course of 2 weeks result in a 60% reduction in the MPD.

Body Site

Palmoplantar skin has a slower rate of absorption as compared with other areas so that the MPD is lowest after a 40 min immersion.

Presence of Disease

Topical psoralen is absorbed more quickly through psoriatic skin as compared with normal skin.

Duration of Photosensitivity

When using a dilute solution of methoxsalen the duration of photosensitivity is short. The MPD is at a minimum in the first 10 min after immersion is greatly increased within an hour, and at 4 hr photosensisivity cannot be detected.

Serum Levels

Methoxsalen is at a very low level or is undetectable in the serum after topical application. In one study, severity of the disease correlated with plasma levels after bath PUVA with detectable levels in half the patients with the most severe disease.

PHOTOBIOLOGY

Action Spectrum

The action spectrum for topical methoxsalen photosensitivity is maximal at 330 nm but there is broad photoreactivity from 313 to 350 nm. This broad action spectrum probably explains why narrow-band (311 nm) radiation and broad-band UVA lamps have similar efficacy in psoriasis in combination with methoxsalen bath treatment.

Time Course of Erythema

Erythema after exposure to a dilute solution of methoxsalen and UVA radiation appears at about 24 hr after exposure and peaks at about 120 hr, about a day later than is seen with oral PUVA.

PATIENT SELECTION

The indications and contraindications for topical PUVA therapy are essentially the same as those for oral PUVA therapy. The patient or the physician may have a preference for topical PUVA therapy in certain situations (Table 2).

TREATMENT SCHEDULES

There are no established protocols for topical PUVA therapy and instead there are various published procedures, some of which have been studied in some detail. There are two sources of methoxsalen: Oxsoralen lotion

Table 2 Preference for Topical vs. Oral PUVA Therapy

Fear of oral medications
Marked symptoms from oral methoxsalen
Dislike of long treatments, e.g., skin types IV–VI
Potential psoralen–drug interactions, e.g., Phenobarbital
Marked hepatic dysfunction

Table 3   Bath PUVA Therapy

Bathe in a dilute methoxsalen solution at 37°C immersed up to the neck for 15 min
Pat dry
Immediate exposure to UVA radiation
Frequency: two or three times a week

1% (70% alcohol, propylene glycol, acetone, and water) and Oxsoralen
Ultra 10 mg capsules (alcohol solution in a soft gelatin capsule).

Bath PUVA

The general outline of the treatment is given in Table 3.

Methoxsalen Concentration

A wide range of concentrations have been used and there are no comparative studies. For a low-dose schedule a 0.5 mg/L final concentration in bath
water appears to be effective (Table 4). This can be achieved by heating five
capsules in three cups of water in a microwave oven until the gelatin
dissolves or using 5 mL of the Oxsoralen 1% (10 mg/mL) lotion and adding
to 100 L of bath water. For a high-dose schedule (Table 5) 30 mL of the
Oxsoralen lotion is added to 100 L of bath water to give a final concentration of 3 mg/mL.

A word of caution: when preparing or handling methoxsalen solutions, the operator must wear gloves and the patient must avoid splashing
bath water on previously nonexposed areas.

Doses of UVA Radiation

The initial dose is best determined by measuring the MPD. A suitable range
of testing dosages for the low-dose schedule (Table 4) is 1.0, 2.0, 4.0, 6.0, 8.0,
10.0, 12.0, and 14.0 J/cm^2. A suitable range for the high-dose schedule

Table 4   Low-Dose Methoxsalen PUVA Bath Protocol

---

50 mg of methoxsalen dissolved in 100 L of bath water agitated to ensure even
  dispersion
Initial UVA dose determined by
  MPD
    40% of MPD
  Skin type
    1 J/cm^2 for I and II
    2 J/cm^2 for III and IV
    3 J/cm^2 for V and VI
Increase in UVA dose by 1 J/cm^2 each treatment starting at treatment 3 or 5

Table 5 High-Dose Methoxsalen PUVA Bath Protocol

---

300 mg of methoxsalen in 100 L of bath water agitated to ensure even dispersion
Initial UVA dose determined by
  MPD
    40% of MPD
  Skin type
    0.2 J/cm² for I and II
    0.4 J/cm² for II and III
    0.6 J/cm² for IV–VI
Increase UVA dose by half of initial dose each treatment starting at treatment 3 or 5

(Table 5) is 0.5, 1.0, 1.5, 2.0, 2.5, 3.0, 4.0, and 5 J/cm². Alternatively, initial doses of UVA radiation can be determined by skin typing as outlined in the tables.

Soak PUVA

This term is used to describe a topical therapy for treatment of disease on the palms and soles and the protocols used have been similar to those for bath PUVA. Usually, a basin capable of holding about 5 L of water is used and concentrations of methoxsalen ranging from 0.5 mg/L and above have been employed. With soak PUVA it is especially important not to allow the solution to splash onto previously nonexposed areas.

Cream and Gel PUVA

Methoxsalen has been used in cream and gel bases to treat local and more extensive disease with good preliminary results. The kinetics of photosensitivity are similar to bath PUVA, irradiation is performed immediately after removal of the cream, and photosensitivity is lost within 2 hr. Hyperpigmentation was not a problem.

Lotion PUVA

Direct application of Oxsoralen lotion to plaques of psoriasis is not an acceptable treatment. This form of PUVA produces prolonged photosensitivity, which can last a week or more, a high frequency of bullous erythemal reactions, and intense pigmentation that can persist for a year or more.

PRECAUTIONS

The precautions required with topical PUVA therapy are essentially the same as those for oral PUVA, with minor variations. Following bath or soak PUVA therapy, 4 hrs of avoidance of sun exposure appear to be adequate. Eye protection is a debatable issue. From a scientific viewpoint it is probably unnecessary. From a medico-legal viewpoint it should be used since detectable serum levels are found in some patients.

SIDE EFFECTS

Short-Term

Phototoxicity is the main adverse effect reported in studies and its frequency depends on the aggressiveness of the treatment protocol. Erythema, pruritus, and pain are similar in duration to that seen with oral PUVA. Gastrointestinal disturbances and central nervous system symptoms are not seen with topical PUVA therapy.

Long-Term

There is no information on the long-term safety of topical methoxsalen PUVA therapy. Because of the very low serum levels that occur with topical PUVA therapy, the potential risk of cataracts should be nonexistent.

ADVANTAGES/DISADVANTAGES OF TOPICAL PUVA THERAPY

The relative advantages and disadvantages of topical PUVA therapy is a much debated issue with some people taking an almost evangelical approach to the issue. This debate does lead to some confusion at times even though the facts are fairly plain.

Advantages

Five advantages are usually raised, two are true and the other three are fallacious.

Reduced Systemic Exposure to Methoxsalen

The greatly reduced levels of methoxsalen in serum and in eyes resulting from topical methoxsalen therapy is a clear advantage of this treatment. Gastrointestinal disturbances, central nervous system symptoms, and cataracts are virtually eliminated as problems.

Reduced Duration of Photosensitivity

The precaution of avoiding exposure to sunlight is only necessary for about 2 hrs after treatment as compared to the remainder of the day with oral PUVA therapy.

Improved Efficacy

There is no evidence that topical PUVA therapy is superior in efficacy to oral PUVA therapy. The aggressiveness of dosimetry in respect of drug and radiation determines efficacy; an aggressive topical PUVA protocol will be more effective than a conservative oral PUVA protocol and vice versa.

Reduced Risk of Skin Cancer

There is no information on the potential carcinogenicity of topical methoxsalen PUVA therapy in humans. The confusion here has been introduced by reports from Scandinavia that trimethylpsoralen bath therapy is not associated with an increased risk of skin cancer as compared to the increased risk associated with oral methoxsalen PUVA therapy. This may be explained by the finding in mice that topical trimethylpsoralen is less carcinogenic than topical methoxsalen. However, using the same mouse study as a guide there is no reason to expect that oral and topical methoxsalen therapy have different cancer risks.

Reduced Exposure to UVA Radiation

The exposure dose of UVA radiation is low if a high concentration of methoxsalen is used but, except for patient comfort, this is an irrelevant issue since it is probably the number of adducts formed in DNA that determines the therapeutic effect and long-term side effects. For a given MPD, a high concentration of psoralen in the skin combined with a low dose of radiation will result in the same number of cross-links in DNA as will a low concentration of psoralen combined with a high dose of radiation.

Disadvantages

There appear to be two disadvantages in using topical or bath PUVA therapy and they mainly impact physicians in the United States.

Cost

Topical methoxsalen PUVA therapy is much more costly to provide because bathing facilities have to be available, the overall treatment takes longer and more methoxsalen may be used. Unless the patient lives close by, baths have to be available in the office because photosensitivity declines rapidly. This has obvious economic, logistical, and sanitary implications. More space is required and additional staff is needed to supervise the bathing and clean the tub between patients. If high-dose methoxsalen baths are used, the cost of the drug alone is over $100 for each bath.

Medico-Legal Issues

When Oxsoralen lotion is used as a source of methoxsalen for bath and soak PUVA therapy this probably is consistent with customary and ordinary clinical practice provided it is done under the direct supervision of the physician. When Oxsoralen capsules are used as a source of methoxsalen, it is a totally different issue. Oxsoralen capsules are approved for swallowing, not for cutting open or heating and our lawyer friends have frequently focused on this as being a most uncustomary clinical practice. When a disgruntled patient suffers an adverse effect such as a phototoxic erythema, which will occur in about 10% of patients treated with soak or bath PUVA therapy, a lawyer will not be interested in why it occurred but instead on how it occurred.

OTHER FORMS OF TOPICAL THERAPY

Bath Methoxsalen/311 nm Radiation

Using a high dose of methoxsalen (3 mg/mL) in bath water and subsequent exposure to 311 nm narrow-band radiation or broad-band UVA radiation, narrow-band radiation was found to be superior in clearing psoriasis.

Trimethypsoralen Bath Therapy

This form of topical therapy is most widely used in Scandinavia and is very effective in clearing psoriasis. One disadvantage of the treatment is that photosensitivity persists for up to 48 hr, so protection and avoidance of exposure to sunlight are required throughout the clearance course of treatment.

5-Methoxypsoralen Bath Therapy

Similar rates have been reported for 5-methoxypsoralen as compared to methoxsalen using bath therapy for clearance of psoriasis.

BIBLIOGRAPHY

Reviews and Guidelines

Halpern SM, Anstey AV, Dawe RS, Diffey BL, Farr PM, Ferguson J, Hawk JLM, Ibbotson S, McGregor JM, Murphy GM, Thomas SE, Rhodes LE. Guidelines for topical PUVA: a report of a workshop of the British Photodermatology Group. Br J Dermatol 2000; 142:22–31.

Lüftl M, Degitz K, Plewig G, Röcken M. Psoralen bath plus UV-A therapy. Arch Dermatol 1997; 133:1597–1603.

Morison WL. Variations of PUVA: practical and effective? Arch Dermatol 1998; 134:1286–1288.

Pharmacology and Photobiology

Azurdia RM, Dean MP, Rhodes LE. Reduction in 8-methoxypsoralen immersion time alters the erythemal response to bath PUVA. Photodermatol Photoimmunol Photomed 2000; 16:186–188.

Gruss C, Behrens S, von Kobyletzki G, Reuther T, Husebo L, Altmeyer P, Kerscher M. Effects of water temperature on photosensitization in bath-PUVA therapy with 8-methoxypsoralen. Photodermatol Photoimmunol Photomed 1998; 14:145–147.

Calzavara-Pinton PG, Ortel B, Carlino AM, Hönigsmann H, De Panfilis G. Phototesting and phototoxic side effects in bath PUVA. J Am Acad Dermatol 1993; 28:657–659.

Cripps DJ, Lowe NJ, Lerner AB. Action spectra of topical psoralens: a re-evaluation. Br J Dermatol 1982; 107:77–82.

Dolezal E, Seeber A, Hönigsmann H, Tanew A. Correlation between bathing time and photosensitivity in 8-methoxypsoralen (8-MOP) bath PUVA. Photodermatol Photoimmunol Photomed 2000; 16:183–185.

Gómez MI, Azaña JM, Arranz I, Harto A, Ledo A. Plasma levels of 8-methoxypsoralen after bath-PUVA for psoriasis: relationship to disease severity. Br J Dermatol 1995; 133:37–40.

Gruss C, Behrens S, Reuther T, Husebo L, Neumann N, Altmeyer P, Lehmann P, Kerscher M. Kinetics of photosensitivity in bath-PUVA photochemotherapy. J Am Acad Dermatol 1998; 39:443–446.

Hallman CP, Koo JYM, Omohundro C, Lee J. Plasma levels of 8-methoxypsoralen after topical paint PUVA on nonpalmoplantar psoriatic skin. J Am Acad Dermatol 1994; 31:273–275.

von Kobyletzki G, Hoffman K, Kerscher M, Altmeyer P. Plasma levels of 8-methoxypsoralen following PUVA-bath photochemotherapy. Photodermatol Photoimmunol Photomed 1998; 14:136–138.

Konya J, Diffey BL, Hindson TC. Time course of activity of topical 8-methoxypsoralen on palmoplantar skin. Br J Dermatol 1992; 127:654–659.

Koulu LM, Jansén CT. Skin phototoxicity variations during repeated bath PUVA exposures to 8-methoxypsoralen and trimethylpsoralen. Clin Exp Dermatol 1984; 9:64–69.

Man I, Dawe RS, Ferguson J, Ibbotson SH. An intraindividual study of the characteristics of erythema induced by bath and oral methoxsalen photochemotherapy and narrowband ultraviolet B. Photochem Photobiol 2003; 78(1):55–60.

Man I, Dawe RS, Ferguson J, Ibbotson SH. The optimal time to determine the minimal phototoxic dose in skin photosensitized by topical 8 methoxypsoralen. Br J Dermatol 2004; 151:179–182.

Man I, Kwok YK, Dawe RS, Ferguson J, Ibbotson SH. The time course of topical PUVA erythema following 15-and 5-minute methoxsalen immersion. Arch Dermatol 2003; 139:331–334.

Man I, McKinlay J, Dawe RS, Ferguson J, Ibbotson SH. An intraindividual comparative study of psoralen-UVA erythema induced by bath 8-methoxypsoralen and 4, 5', 8-trimethylpsoralen. J Am Acad Dermatol 2003; 49:59–64.

Neumann NJ, Ruzicka T, Lehmann P. Rapid decrease of phototoxicity after PUVA bath therapy with 8-methoxypsoralen. Arch Dermatol 1996; 132:1394.

Schempp CM, Schöpf E, Simon JC. Phototesting in bath-PUVA: marked reduction of 8-methoxypsoralen (8-MOP) activity within one hour after an 8-MOP bath. Photodermatol Photoimmunol Photomed 1996; 12:100–102.

Schiener R, Behrens-Williams SC, Pillekamp H, Peter RU, Kerscher M. Does the minimal phototoxic dose after 8-methoxypsoralen baths correlate with the individual's skin phototype? Photodermatol Photoimmunol Photomed 2001; 17:156–158.

Tanew A, Kipfelsperger T, Seeber A, Radakovic-Fijan S, Hönigsmann H. Correlation between 8-methoxypsoralen bath-water concentration and photosensitivity in bath-PUVA treatment. J Am Acad Dermatol 2001; 44:638–642.

Treatment Protocols

Behrens S, von Kobyletzki G, Gruss C, Reuther T, Altmeyer P, Kerscher M. PUVA-bath photochemotherapy (PUVA-soak therapy) of recalcitrant dermatoses of the palms and soles. Photodermatol Photoimmunol Photomed 1999; 15:47–51.

Calzavara-Pinton PG, Ortel B, Hönigsmann H, Zane C, De Panfilis G. Safety and effectiveness of an aggressive and individualized bath-PUVA regimen in the treatment of psoriasis. Dermatol 1994; 189:256–259.

Coleman WR, Lowe NJ, David M, Halder RM. Palmoplantar psoriasis: experience with 8-methoxypsoralen soaks plus ultraviolet A with the use of a high-output metal halide device. J Am Acad Dermatol 1989; 20:1078–1082.

Collins P, Rogers S. Bath-water compared with oral delivery of 8-methoxypsoralen PUVA therapy for chronic plaque psoriasis. Br J Dermatol 1992; 127:392–395.

Gange RW, Levins P, Murray J, Anderson RR, Parrish JA. Prolonged skin photosensitization induced by methoxsalen and subphototoxic UVA irradiation. J Invest Dermatol 1984; 82:219–222.

Grundmann-Kollmann M, Tegeder I, Ochsendorf FR, Zollner TM, Ludwig R, Kaufmann R, Podda M. Kinetics and dose-response of photosensitivity in cream psoralen plus ultraviolet A photochemotherapy: comparative *in vivo* studies after topical application of three standard preparations. Br J Dermatol 2001; 144:991–995.

Lowe NJ, Weingarten D, Bourget T, Moy LS. PUVA therapy for psoriasis: comparison of oral and bath-water delivery of 8-methoxypsoralen. J Am Acad Dermataol 1986; 14:754–760.

Simons JR, Bohnen IJWE, Van Der Valk PGM. A left-right comparison of UVB phototherapy and topical photochemotherapy in bilateral chronic hand dermatitis after 6 weeks' treatment. Clin Exp Dermatol 1997; 22:7–10.

de Rie MA, Van Eendenburg JP, Versnick AC, Stolk LML, Bos JD, Westerhof W. A new psoralen-containing gel for topical PUVA therapy: development, and treatment results in patients with palmoplantar and plaque-type psoriasis, and hyperkeratotic eczema. Br J Dermatol 1995; 132:964–969.

Schempp CM, Müller H, Czech W, Schöpf E, Simon JC. Treatment of chronic palmoplantar eczema with local bath-PUVA therapy. J Am Acad Dermatol 1997; 36:733–737.

Vallat VP, Gilleaudeau P, Battat L, Wolfe J, Heftler N, Gottlieb SL, Hodak E, Gottlieb AB, Krueger JG. PUVA bath therapy with 8-methoxypsoralen. In: Weinstein GD, Gottlieb AB, eds. Therapy of Moderate-to-Severe Psoriasis, Stanford, CT: Haber and Flora, Inc.,1993:39–55.

Other Forms of Topical Therapy

Hannuksela M, Karvonen J. Trioxsalen bath plus UVA effective and safe in the treatment of psoriasis. Br J Dermatol 1978; 99:703–707.

Hannuksela A, Pukkala E, Hannuksela M, Karvonen J. Cancer incidence among Finnish patients with psoriasis treated with trioxsalen bath PUVA. J Am Acad Dermatol 1996; 35:685–689.

Väätäinen N. Phototoxicity of topical trioxsalen. Arch Dermatovener (Stockh) 1980; 60:327–331.

Ortel B, Perl S, Kinaciyan T, Calzavara-Pinton PG, Hönigsmann H. Comparison of narrow-band (311 nm) UVB and broad-band UVA after oral or bath-water 8-methoxypsoralen in the treatment of psoriasis. J Am Acad Dermatol 1993; 29:736–740.

11

UVB Phototherapy

INTRODUCTION

Strictly speaking there is no such thing as "UVB" phototherapy since there are no radiation sources with an emission spectrum restricted to the UVB waveband and all emit longer and shorter wavelengths. However, wavelengths in the UVB waveband are responsible for most of the therapeutic effect.

Two types of UVB phototherapy are available: narrowband and broadband and the principles underlying these treatments and protocols used are different, therefore they will be discussed separately. However other aspects of the treatments such as adjunctive treatment, maintenance, adverse effects, and protection are similar and will be addressed collectively.

THE TREATMENTS

Narrowband UVB Phototherapy

Background

Narrowband UVB phototherapy has also been called selective UV therapy and 311 nm UV therapy because the fluorescent bulb used in the treatment has a narrow emission spectrum which peaks at 311 nm. The principle underlying this treatment is that the longer UVB wavelengths are more therapeutic and much less erythemogenic than wavelengths below 300 nm. An elegant study by Parrish and Jaenicke, extending a previous study by

Fischer, has placed that hypothesis on a scientific footing by accurately defining the action spectrum for phototherapy of psoriasis. Wavelengths shorter than 295 nm had minimal or no detectable therapeutic effect; these wavelengths are very effective in producing erythema of normal skin. Wavelengths longer than 295 nm were more therapeutic and less erythemogenic. For example, monochromatic 313 nm radiation cleared psoriasis in doses as low as 0.2 × MED. These findings indicated that a radiation source with a predominant emission in the 300–320 nm waveband might be very effective in the treatment of psoriasis.

These observations resulted in the development and use of a lamp made by Philips, a European lighting company, which was found to be clearly superior to broadband therapy using the sunlamp fluorescent bulb.

Narrowband UVB therapy quickly replaced the older treatments in Europe but was introduced in the United States in the mid-1990s only. There were several reasons for this slow introduction. First, the bulbs are an inch longer than those in use here, and therefore did not fit in existing units. Second, to keep the duration of a treatment short, a dedicated unit containing 48 narrowband bulbs is ideal as compared to the eight broadband bulbs in older combination units. Third, the bulbs are very expensive and have a much shorter effective lifespan as compared to sunlamp bulbs. These practical and economic disincentives to using the treatment have resulted in a gradual, rather than rapid increase in the availability of this treatment.

Protocols

A commonly used protocol for the treatment is outlined in Table 1. MED testing is an essential first step for controlled and effective treatment (see Chapter 5). This protocol is aimed at being suberythemogenic but erythema is likely to occur under three circumstances. First, in people with skin types I and II, if treatments are given on consecutive days erythema is likely to occur and the dose should not be raised for the second of two consecutive

Table 1   Treatment Protocol for Narrowband Phototherapy

Test MED
Read MED at 24 hr, give first whole-body treatment at 70% MED, consider extra to
    limbs at 35% MED
Treat Monday, Wednesday, Friday, increase dose 10% each treatment
If erythema occurs
    Asymptomatic: hold dose
    Symptomatic but has subsided: reduce dose by 20%
    Symptomatic and still present: withhold treatment and reduce dose 20% for next
        treatment

Table 2 Schedule for Treatment Interruptions

Dose adjustments depend on duration of absence
1 week: hold at previous dose
2 weeks: reduce dose by 25%
3 weeks: reduce dose by 50%
4 weeks: restart at beginning of schedule

treatments. Second, almost all patients will reach their erythema threshold during a course of treatment, and this usually necessitates holding the dose at a fixed level thereafter. Third, tolerance is lost fairly quickly, so if treatment is interrupted the guidelines outlined in Table 2 should be followed. It is a wise move to warn patients of these risks of erythema at the time of initiating treatment so that they will not be surprised when it occurs.

Some variations of this protocol have been used. More aggressive dose increments of 20% or more have been reported, but this is likely to be associated with more frequent erythemas. A twice weekly schedule has been reported as effective; but this slows down the response and results in fewer patients reaching adequate clearance of disease. Note that a schedule of four or five treatments a week provides clearance with fewer treatments, but in the same number of days due to frequent delays caused by erythemas.

When there is significant disease on the limbs an extra exposure to limbs only may be given, starting at half the whole-body dose and increasing 10% per treatment. Narrowband therapy is not therapeutic for disease on the palms and soles in patients above the age of about 10 years. The reason is simple: an adequate dose of UVB radiation does not penetrate the thicker epidermis at these sites. In young children a response is sometimes seen on the palms and soles.

Skin typing can be used as an alternative to MED testing to determine the initial exposure dose. Obviously, this approach has to be used in patients with very extensive disease and insufficient skin to phototest. Suggested starting doses by skin type are listed in Table 3. The main problem with this

Table 3 Initial Exposure Dose by Skin Typing for Narrowband Phototherapy

Skin type	Dose (mJ/cm^2)
I	300
II	400
III	600
IV	800
V	1000
VI	1500

approach is that there is a poor correlation between skin type and MED so that underdosing or overdosing is likely to occur. If the dose selected is well below the MED, treatments are wasted and the chance of successful clearance is reduced because of excessive tanning. Selection of a dose that is too high increases the risk of erythema.

Results of Treatment

Most studies report clearance rates (< 95% of original disease) of about 80% of unselected patients when treatments are given three times each week. This number drops to about 60% when using a schedule of two treatments each week. There are reports that narrowband UVB is as effective as PUVA therapy but such findings must be viewed with some reservation. Patients with thick plaques, very inflammatory disease, and very extensive disease respond more readily to PUVA therapy. In addition, there are quite a few patients who do not clear with narrowband treatment and subsequently clear with PUVA therapy.

Broadband UVB Phototherapy

Background

During a series of studies investigating the efficacy of various components of the Goeckerman regimen, it was found that high-dose UVB phototherapy using sunlamp bulbs (broadband UVB) was an effective treatment in many patients with psoriasis. High dose in this context means using a treatment schedule aimed at staying close to or above the erythema threshold of the patient throughout the course of treatment. The dose regimens have been developed empirically and, because of individual variation, will not be ideal for all patients. Therefore, close supervision of patients, accurate radiometry, and well-trained staff are essential. In short, broadband UVB phototherapy is probably the most difficult UV treatment to deliver in a successful manner.

The Treatment

Explanation to the patient: High-dose UVB phototherapy is a treatment that produces an adverse effect, namely erythema, in all patients. Therefore, this has to be explained to the patient. It must be emphasized that

- The production of erythema is an aim of the treatment and without this effect, treatment is unlikely to be successful.
- Mild erythema, pink without significant discomfort, is likely to follow as many as half of all the treatments.
- Symptomatic erythema will occur at least once during any course of treatment. The production of erythema is not an exact science, and over- and undershooting are common.

Table 4 Treatment Protocol for Broadband UVB Phototherapy

Test MED

Read MED at 24 hr, give first whole-body treatment at 70% MED, consider adding
  extra to limbs at 35% MED

Treat three, four, or five times a week, increase dose 20% each treatment

If erythema occurs

  Asymptomatic: hold dose

  Symptomatic but has subsided: reduce dose by 10%

  Symptomatic and still present: withhold treatment and reduce doses for next
    treatment by 10%

The development of erythema should not be regarded as a side effect
of the therapy but as an essential component and a sign that the treatment is
likely to be successful. If this positive attitude is conveyed to the patient with
a frank admission that symptomatic erythema is inevitable, patients will
accept the problem without complaint.

Protocols: Various schedules have been used for broadband UVB
phototherapy and the one outlined in Table 4 is effective and fairly simple.
The initial determination of the MED is essential for controlled treatment.
Another essential component is that the treatment must be given at least
three times a week since a twice weekly schedule is seldom successful. Four
or five treatments each week are even more preferable, particularly in skin
types III and higher.

If there is significant disease on the limbs, extra treatment for those
areas is required from the time the therapy begins; an additional 50% of
the whole-body dose should be given after covering the trunk and face.
After 15–20 treatments, symptomatic erythema can become troublesome,
and the increment to the whole-body dose should be reduced to 10% for
each treatment when this occurs.

Broadband phototherapy shares two features with narrowband phototherapy, which have already been mentioned. Tolerance to therapy is
rapidly lost so that if treatment is interrupted the same dose schedule
outlined in Table 2 should be followed. Broadband phototherapy is not
effective for disease on the palms and soles in most patients.

Results of Treatment

In unselected patients treated with broadband UVB therapy about 60% will
achieve clearance to < 95% of the original disease. Selection of patients who
have a short history, moderate disease, thin plaques, and a good response to
sunlight can push the response rate above 80%. Broadband UVB phototherapy is clearly not as effective as narrowband UVB phototherapy and it is a

more difficult treatment to administer. Consequently, it is likely to be gradually phased out.

ADJUNCTIVE TREATMENT

The only topical medication required is the application of an emollient before exposure to radiation. Any lubricant will suffice as long as it makes the psoriatic scale transparent (see Fig. 1). The importance of this aspect of the treatment is greatest in the early phase of clearance therapy when psoriatic scale is obviously present. However, it should be continued until full clearance has been achieved. Free use of lubricants is permitted at other times of the day. Calcipotriene, tar, salicylic acid, and anthralin should not be applied before treatment since they absorb UVB radiation and reduce the efficacy of treatment.

The scalp, in a person with hair at that site, and intertriginous areas do require some adjunctive therapy since UVB phototherapy does not have a systemic effect, and these sites are shielded from exposure. Suitable topical therapy or excimer laser treatment should be considered.

RESPONSE TO THERAPY

The sequence of changes observed in psoriatic plaques responding to UVB phototherapy is decreased scaling and decreased thickness of the plaques, so that only macular erythema remains at the site of the plaque. This erythema is gradually replaced by normal or increased pigmentation of the skin. While

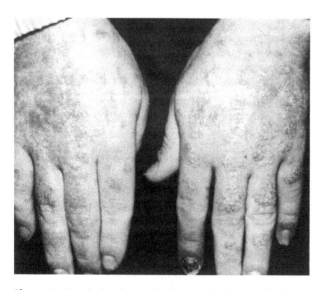

Figure 1 Psoriatic plaques before and after application of a lubricant. Note the apparent disappearance of scale.

erythema persists, a biopsy will still show evidence of psoriasis, and it is important not to accept erythema as an end point of treatment since a rapid recurrence of disease will occur. It is also important for the therapist to know, and to make the patient aware, that the actual size of the plaques does not diminish during the phase of resolution, i.e., plaques do not resolve by shrinkage. Success of treatment is indicated by some obvious change in the plaques by 10 treatments and clearance of disease to >95% of the original involvement should occur by 30 treatments. However, in clinical practice outside a trial, clearance may require as few as 10 treatments, or as many as 60 treatments.

The duration of the remission, after a successful clearance course of treatment without maintenance, averages less than 3 months and this is much shorter than with PUVA therapy.

MAINTENANCE THERAPY

Following the introduction of PUVA therapy, attention has been given to the desirability of maintaining patients in a relatively disease-free condition over long periods. Certainly, patients like to be free of disease. UVB phototherapy can include a maintenance phase, and this has been shown to significantly prolong the duration of remission (Table 5). However, only about 30% of patients can maintain control of their disease with weekly therapy, and the remainder require either twice weekly or alternating weekly/twice weekly treatments

There are several problems with using UVB phototherapy as a maintenance treatment:

- The high frequency of treatment, i.e., four to eight treatments each month, becomes too time-consuming for many patients, and they simply stop treatment.
- Patients with skin types I and II begin to have a significant loss of tolerance to UV radiation after 7 days, presumably due to loss of tan and thickening of the stratum corneum, so that erythema becomes a problem. This particularly occurs if the patient is scheduling weekly treatments on the basis of calendar weeks, so that a

Table 5 Maintenance Treatment Schedule for UVB Phototherapy

Reduce to BIW schedule for 4 weeks, hold dose at level of last clearance treatment
If no recurrence, reduce to QW schedule
If significant recurrence occurs on maintenance:
   Return to TIW schedule until controlled
   Then reduce to BIW and QW as before
   Consider alternating QW/BIW schedule

treatment may be given on a Monday and then the next treatment is received 11 days later on the Friday of the next week. To overcome these deficiencies of UVB phototherapy as a maintenance program it has been suggested that patients be switched to PUVA therapy for maintenance. This is a good idea, in principle, but it has not been very successful since it is difficult to select the correct dose that will control the disease and not produce erythema.

PRECAUTIONS

During Treatment

1. The eyes must be protected with UV-opaque goggles during exposure in the treatment unit. An occasional exception may be made in patients with recalcitrant disease of the eyelids or periorbital skin at the discretion of the physician.
2. The face, genitalia in men, and sunlight- or radiation-damaged skin should be shielded unless involved with significant disease. The face already receives the highest exposure dose of UVB radiation from sunlight and there is no need to give it additional exposure.

Before and After Treatment

1. Patients should avoid additional exposure to UVB radiation in sunlight during the course of treatment. On the day of treatment, this should be rigorously adhered to because the patient has already received a potentially erythemogenic dose, and additional outdoor exposure could lead to a severe sunburn. On nontreatment days, sunbathing will induce pigmentation and thus reduce the effectiveness of treament.
2. Patients should be encouraged to use sunscreen on exposed areas at all times.

ADVERSE EFFECTS

UVB phototherapy has both short-term and long-term risks and, as previously mentioned, warning patients about the common ones is an important first step in managing these problems (Table 6).

Short-Term Side Effects

Phototoxicity in the skin accounts for almost all of the short-term problems of the therapy and other problems are rare.

Table 6 Side Effects of UVB Phototherapy

Short-term
  The skin
    Erythema
    Pruritus
    Bullae on psoriatic plaques
    Subacute phototoxicity
    New rash (see "Problem Cases," Chapter
      20)
    The eye
      Blepharitis
    Infections
      Recurrent herpes labialis
    Autoimmune disorders
      Lupus erythematosus
      Pemphigus
      Pemphigoid
Long-term
    Photoaging
    Nonmelanoma skin cancer
    Immunosuppression

The Skin

Erythema: The main short-term problem is erythema and this is usually of short duration. It is a central component of broadband UVB therapy and it will occur at least once during a course of narrowband UVB treatment. The main elements of management of a symptomatic erythema are listed in Table 7. It is very important for the physician and staff to keep focused on the fact that this is a sunburn, just the same as the sunburns people develop when they stay out in the sun during summer, and there will be no long-term consequences. Problems often arise when patients visit an emergency room or 24 hr clinic and are told they have a second-degree burn. Such terminology applies to thermal burns, which of course can scar. Problems can be averted by making sure the patient is seen, managed correctly, educated, and followed.

There are several treatments that should not be used in the management of UVB-induced erythema. Topical and oral corticosteroids do not influence the course of the erythema; topical steroids will act as moisturizers and oral steroids may make the patient happier but there is no specific effect. Similarly, NSAIDs do not affect the course of the erythema. Topical anesthetics containing benzocaine should not be used because they have a high rate of sensitization and a contact dermatitis will only further complicate the situation.

Table 7 Management of Symptomatic UVB-Induced Erythema

Always see and evaluate the patient
Attempt to find the cause
Provide regular follow-up until settled
If localized, may continue treatment while shielding the area with zinc oxide or
  clothing
If widespread, stop therapy and use symptomatic measures: moisturizers, cool
  oatmeal baths, and analgesics such as aspirin and acetominophen
Treatments to avoid include topical and oral corticosteroids, NSAIDs, and
  benzocaine anesthetics

It is always important to try and determine the cause of a symptomatic erythema. The best place to start is the flow sheet since missed treatments are a leading cause of erythema. The staff should have noted that treatments had been missed and adjusted the dose accordingly but, of course, this is not always the case and patients may not volunteer the information because of forgetfulness or guilt about not coming for treatment. A common cause of a local erythema, for example, confined to the head and neck or over the breasts and buttocks, is that the patient forgot to shield those areas as they had been doing for all previous treatments.

Pruritus: Dryness of the skin is the usual cause of pruritus and this can be avoided and treated by frequent lubrication. Pruritus may also be an early warning of phototoxicity.

Bullae on psoriatic plaques: A rare problem is the development of blisters on psoriatic plaques. This may be due to excessive phototoxicity, but it is usually not associated with erythema of the surrounding normal skin. The possibility of pemphigoid or pemphigus must be considered, although we have not found this to be the cause in affected patients.

Subacute phototoxicity: This is also a rare problem but I have seen two patients develop this problem while being treated with narrowband phototherapy. The clinical picture was identical to that seen in PUVA patients (see Chapter 9) with sudden onset of pruritus and a psoriasiform eruption.

The Eye

Blepharitis is an occasional problem when a patient forgets to use goggles while in the unit. A consultation with an opthalmologist is a wise precaution but treatment is symptomatic and the condition settles fairly quickly.

Infections

The frequency of recurrent herpes labialis is probably increased, but primary infection does not appear to be more common.

Autoimmunity

Lupus erythematosus, pemphigus, and bullous pemphigoid can all be experimentally induced by exposure to UVB radiation in patients with a predisposition to these diseases, so they are theoretical risks of the treatment. However, they do not appear to have been reported and hence must be very rare.

Long-Term Side Effects

UVB phototherapy is usually considered to be associated with minimal long-term risk. This comfortable and happy perception may be true but there are four provisos that should be considered before accepting this position.

- Exposure to UVB radiation is clearly established as causing photoaging, nonmelanoma skin cancer, and immunosuppression in experimental animals and these effects are dose-dependent.
- Exposure to sunlight is clearly established as causing photoaging, nonmelanoma skin cancer, and immunosuppression in humans, and people with skin types I and II are most susceptible to these effects. The UVB component of sunlight is generally accepted to be the major cause of these problems.
- Until quite recently, most exposure to UVB phototherapy has consisted of short, intermittent courses of treatment, as, for example, a Goeckerman program for 3 weeks, once or twice a year. UVB phototherapy with continued maintenance results in a much higher exposure dose.
- Finally, there are no prospective studies on the long-term risks of UVB phototherapy. We should always remember the maxim: what you do not look for you will not find. If long-term studies of PUVA therapy had not been conducted, a possible association of melanoma with this treatment would not be suspected, and firm evidence of the increased risk of nonmelanoma skin cancer would have been delayed for many years.

Photoaging

Increased freckling is seen in patients who have been treated with long courses of both broadband and narrowband phototherapy. This is most evident in skin types I and II and does not appear to occur in higher skin types. However, there are no published studies of freckling or other signs of photoaging in patients treated with UVB phototherapy. The relative contribution of sunlight exposure, frequently used by the same patients as a therapy, is also unknown.

Skin Cancer

Bearing in mind what is known from studies in mice and the effect of sunlight on humans, it would be anticipated that exposure to broadband UVB phototherapy is associated with an increased risk of nonmelanoma skin cancer; this possibility has been the subject of only a few studies in humans. A potential problem in such studies is that most psoriatic patients have also been treated with tar, a well-known carcinogen, in addition to broadband UVB radiation, so that it is difficult to determine the relative importance of the two agents. In one study, exposure of patients with psoriasis to tar and UVB radiation was found to be associated with an increased incidence of skin cancer, but in another study, the incidence was similar to that in the general population. A different approach gave an estimate that patients treated with high-dose UVB phototherapy with maintenance treatment have a risk of developing skin cancer that is 2.5–7.5 times the risk in outdoor workers. This calculation was based on epidemiologic data, and studies in animals. Review of these limited data and known exposure doses leads to the conclusion that broadband UVB phototherapy is probably associated with an increased risk of nonmelanoma skin cancer and when maintenance therapy is provided, either in the office or at home, this increased risk is probably substantial.

The potential for narrowband UVB radiation to cause nonmelanoma skin cancer is even more uncertain. There are no studies in humans of its carcinogenic potential; so for the foreseeable future we must rely on data from mouse and in vitro studies. Narrowband UVB is two to three times more carcinogenic than broadband UVB in mice when they are exposed to equi-erythemogenic doses. When the same ratio of doses are applied to human cells in vitro, a similar number of "direct hit" lesions are produced in DNA for both wavebands but narrowband UVB produces more oxygen-mediated DNA damage. Some people have questioned the relevance of these findings to clinical practice since narrowband UVB therapy usually involves a lower exposure in terms of the number of MEDs. Probably a middle-of-the-road comment would be: we don't know but narrowband UVB therapy is likely to be as carcinogenic as broadband UVB therapy, if not more so, but both are less carcinogenic than PUVA therapy.

Immunosuppression

UVB phototherapy is immunosuppressive in both animals, such as mice and guinea pigs, and in humans, but there is no evidence that this is relevant as an adverse effect in patients on therapy.

BIBLIOGRAPHY

Narrowband UVB Therapy

Background

Fischer T, Alsins J, Berne B. Ultraviolet-action spectrum and evaluation of ultraviolet lamps for psoriasis healing. Int J Dermatol 1984; 23:633–637.

Ibbotson SH, Bilsland D, Cox NH, Dawe RS, Diffey B, Edwards C, Farr PM, Ferguson J, Hart G, Hawk J, Lloyd J, Martin C, Moseley H, McKenna K, Rhodes LE, Taylor DK. An update and guidance on narrowband ultraviolet B phototherapy: a British Photodermatology Group Workshop report. Br J Dermatol 2004; 151:283–297.

Parrish JA, Jaenicke KF. Action spectrum for phototherapy of psoriasis. J Invest Dermatol 1981; 76:359–362.

Protocols

Cameron H, Dawe RS, Yule S, Murphy J, Ibbotson SH, Ferguson J. A randomized, observer-blinded trial of twice vs. three times weekly narrowband ultraviolet B phototherapy for chronic plaque psoriasis. Br J Dermatol 2002; 147:973–978.

Coven TR, Burack LH, Gilleaudeau P, Keogh M, Ozawa M, Krueger JG. Narrowband UV-B produces superior clinical and histopathological resolution of moderate-to-severe psoriasis in patients compared with broadband UV-B. Arch Dermatol 1997; 133:1514–1522.

Das S, Lloyd JJ, Farr PM. Similar dose-response and persistence of erythema with broad-band and narrow-band ultraviolet B lamps. J Invest Dermatol 2001; 117:1318–1321.

Dawe RS, Wainwright NJ, Cameron H, Ferguson J. Narrow-band (TL-01) ultraviolet B phototherapy for chronic plaque psoriasis: three times or five times weekly treatment? Br J Dermatol 1998; 138:833–839.

Dawe RS, Cameron H, Yule S, Man I, Wainwright NJ, Ibbotson SH, Ferguson J. A randomized controlled trial of narrowband ultraviolet B vs. bath-psoralen plus ultraviolet A photochemotherapy for psoriasis. Br J Dermatol 2003; 148:1194–1204.

Gloor M, Scherotzke A. Age dependence of ultraviolet light-induced erythema following narrow-band UVB exposure. Photodermatol Photoimmunol Photomed 2002; 18:121–126.

Gordon PM, Diffey BL, Matthews JNS, Farr PM. A randomized comparison of narrow-band TL-01 phototherapy and PUVA photochemotherapy for psoriasis. J Am Acad Dermatol 1999; 41:728–732.

Gordon PM, Saunders PJ, Diffey BL, Farr PM. Phototesting prior to narrowband (TL-01) ultraviolet B phototherapy. Br J Dermatol 1998; 139:811–814.

Green C, Ferguson J, Lakshmipathi T, Johnson BE. 311 nm UVB photo-therapy—an effective treatment for psoriasis. Br J Dermatol 1988; 119:691–696.

Leenutaphong V, Sudtim S. A comparison of erythema efficacy of ultraviolet B irradiation from Philips TL12 and TL01 lamps. Photodermatol Photoimmunol Photomed 1998; 14:112–115.

Man I, Dawe RS, Ferguson J, Ibbotson SH. An intraindividual study of the characteristics of erythema induced by bath and oral methoxsalen photochemotherapy and narrowband ultraviolet B. Photochem Photobiol 2003; 78(1):55–60.

Markham T, Rogers S, Collins P. Narowband UV-B (TL-01) phototherapy vs oral 8-methoxypsoralen psoralen-UV-A for the treatment of chronic plaque psoriasis. Arch Dermatol 2003; 139:325–328.

Picot E, Meunier L, Picot-Debeze MC, Peyron JL, Meynadier J. Treatment of psoriasis with a 311-nm UVB lamp. Br J Dermatol 1992; 127: 509–512.

Tanew A, Radakovic-Fijan S, Schemper M, Hönigsmann H. Narrowband UV-B phototherapy vs. photochemotherapy in the treatment of chronic plaque-type psoriasis. Arch Dermatol 1999; 135:519–524.

Van Weelden H, Baart de la Faille H, Young E, van der Leun JC. A new development in UVB phototherapy of psoriasis. Br J Dermatol 1988; 119:11–19.

Walters IB, Burack LH, Coven TR, Gilleaudeau P, Krueger JG. Suberythemogenic narrow-band UVB is markedly more effective than conventional UVB in treatment of psoriasis vulgaris. J Am Acad Dermatol 1999; 40:893–900

Youn JI, Park JY, Jo SJ, Rim JH, Choe YB. Assessment of the usefulness of skin phototype and skin color as the parameter of cutaneous narrow band UVB sensitivity in psoriasis patients. Photoderm Photoimmunol Photomed 2003; 19:261–264.

Broadband UVB Therapy

Background

LeVine MJ, White HAD, Parrish JA. Components of the Goeckerman regimen. J Invest Dermatol 1979; 73:170–173.

Protocols

Adrian RM, Parrish JA, Momtaz TK, Karlin MJ. Outpatient phototherapy for psoriasis. Arch Dermatol 1981; 117:623–626.

LeVine MJ, Parrish JA. Outpatient phototherapy of psoriasis. Arch Dermatol 1980; 116:552–554.

Stern RS, Armstrong RB, Anderson TF, Bickers DR, Lowe NJ, Harber L, Voorhees J, Parrish JA. Effect of continued ultraviolet B phototherapy on the duration of remission of psoriasis: a randomized study. J Am Acad Dermatol 1986; 15:546–552.

Adjunctive Treatment

Hudson-Peacock MJ, Diffey BL, Farr PM. Photoprotective action of emollients in ultraviolet therapy of psoriasis. Br J Dermatol 1994; 130:361–365.
Lebwohl M, Martinez J, Weber P, DeLuca R. Effects of topical preparations on the erythemogenicity of UVB: implications for psoriasis phototherapy. J Am Acad Dermatol 1995; 32:469–471.

UVB and Skin Cancer

Narrowband UVB Therapy

Budiyanto A, Ueda M, Ueda T, Ichihashi M. Formation of cyclobutane pyrimidine dimers and 8-oxo-, 8-dihydro-2'-deoxyguanosine in mouse and organ-cultured human skin by irradiation with broadband or with narrowband UVB. Photochem Photobiol 2002; 76(4):397–400.
Flindt-Hansen H, McFadden N, Eeg-Larsen T, Thune P. Effect of a new narrow-band UVB lamp on photocarcinogenesis in mice. Acta Dermatol Venereol (Stockh) 1991; 71:245–248.
Gibbs NK, Traynor NJ, MacKie RM, Campbell I, Johnson BE, Ferguson J. The phototumorigenic potential of broad-band (270–350 nm) and narrow-band (311–313 nm) phototherapy sources cannot be predicted by their edematogenic potential in hairless mouse skin. J Invest Dermatol 1995; 104:359–363.
Sterenborg HJCM, van Weelden H, van der Leun JC. The dose-response relationship for tumourigenesis by UV radiation in the region 311–312 nm. J Photochem Photobiol 1988; 2:179–194.
Wulf HC, Hansen AB, Bech-Thomsen M. Differences in narrow-band ultraviolet B and broad-spectrum ultraviolet photocarcinogenesis in lightly pigmented hairless mice. Photodermatol Photoimmunol Photomed 1994; 10:192–197.

Broadband UVB Therapy

Larko O, Swanbeck G. Is UVB treatment of psoriasis safe? A study of extensively UVB-treated psoriasis patients compared with a matched control group. Acta Dermatol Venereol (Stockh) 1982; 62:507–512.
Pitteklow MR, Perry HO, Muller SA, et al. Skin cancer in patients with psoriasis treated with coal tar. Arch Dermatol 1981; 117:465–468.
Schothorst AA, Slaper H, Schouten R, Suurmond D. UVB doses in maintenance psoriasis phototherapy vs. solar UVB exposure. Photodermatology 1985; 2:213–220.

Slaper H, Schothorst AA, van der Leun JC. Risk evaluation of UVB therapy for psoriasis: comparison of calculated risk for UVB therapy and observed risk in PUVA-treated patients. Photodermatology 1986; 3:271–283.

Stern RS, Zierler S, Parrish JA. Skin carcinoma in patients with psoriasis treated with topical tar and artificial ultraviolet radiation. Lancet 1980; i:732–735.

12

Other Forms of Phototherapy

INTRODUCTION

There are several other forms of phototherapy used in the treatment of psoriasis (Table 1) and while these are not widely used, consideration of their advantages and disadvantages is worthwhile.

GOECKERMAN REGIMEN

This treatment is mainly of historic interest now since it is only practiced in a few centers. However, introduction of the treatment in 1925 was a major step forward in the management of psoriasis since it is not only very effective, but in the half century of its widespread use, it also proved to be very safe. At the time of its discovery, Goeckerman was searching for ways to photosensitize the skin and thus increase the therapeutic effectiveness of

Table 1 Other Forms of Phototherapy for Psoriasis

Goeckerman regimen
Tar photosensitization
Home phototherapy
Climatotherapy
Tanning parlor phototherapy

UV radiation. As we will discuss, he discovered the right treatment for the wrong reason.

The Treatment

The two essentials of the treatment are application of crude coal tar in an ointment base and exposure to a source of UV radiation. Many modifications are used. However, a general description of the regimen is that 2–10% crude tar ointment is applied to the plaques of psoriasis or the whole body, excluding the head, neck, and intertriginous areas, one to three times each day. This ointment is partially removed prior to exposure to a source of radiation with the maximal emission in the UVB range. Either a medium-pressure mercury arc lamp or fluorescent sunlamp bulb is most commonly used and the dose of UV radiation is suberythemogenic. Following irradiation, the patient has a tub bath and further ointment is often applied. Mild cases of psoriasis require 2 to 3 weeks of treatment, while severe cases may require 4 or more weeks of this therapy. The overall response rate is high and more than 90% of patients achieve 95% clearance of their disease.

There are many obvious variables in the Goeckerman regimen such as variation in the constituents of crude coal tar depending on the supplier, use of different sources of radiation, and different numbers of application of ointment. In addition, several modifications are often used. Application of topical corticosteroids is often combined with the regimen either initially to reduce inflammation and risk of irritation from the tar or throughout the whole course of treatment. Short-term initial use of these agents may have some benefit. Prolonged use of topical corticosteroids through the whole course of treatment tends to reduce the duration of the subsequent remission without accelerating clearance of disease. Another modification is the use of twice daily exposure to radiation, presumably on the basis of more must be better. However, several studies have found that there is no advantage in using more than one exposure to radiation each day.

Mechanism of the Treatment

The mechanism of action of the Goeckerman regimen has attracted much study and discussion. Tar is definitely therapeutic in psoriasis, but its action is weak, so that this agent alone is seldom effective in clearing disease. UVB radiation is usually given in suberythemogenic doses in the Goeckerman regimen; this alone is therapeutic in psoriasis, but although UVB radiation in these doses is much more therapeutic than tar, again, it is seldom effective in clearing the disease. Therefore, some additive or synergistic effect of tar and UVB radiation must explain the efficacy of the regimen. It was assumed for many years that tar photosensitization was the basis for the interaction of tar and UV radiation. However, this is an unlikely explanation because tar is activated by wavelengths in the UVA waveband. If a sunlamp is used as a source of these wavelengths, UVB phototoxicity in normal skin will greatly exceed UVA-induced tar phototoxicity, or, put in another way, any erythema observed will be due mainly to the effect of UVB radiation.

Recent studies have suggested that application of a tar ointment to the skin may have a synergistic interaction with UVB radiation owing to the effect of the ointment base on the optical properties of psoriatic skin. Plaques of psoriasis are covered with scales separated by air-filled spaces that have a different refractive index than does keratin. Therefore, incident radiation meets multiple optical surfaces so that much of it is scattered and reflected back from the skin. The ointment base, which has a refractive index similar to that of keratin, fills the spaces, reduces scattering, and increases transmission of radiation into the plaque. Therefore, the mechanism of action of the Goeckerman regimen is complex and involves an antimitotic effect of tar, an antimitotic effect of UV radiation, refractive index-matching by the ointment base, and a mild keratolytic effect, also from the base.

Advantages and Disadvantages of the Treatment

There are two advantages of the Goeckerman regimen: it is effective and safe. While these are strong points in its favor, there are some good reasons to question its continued use.

The Treatment is Time-Consuming and Expensive

It was developed as a hospital treatment and only in recent years has it been used in ambulatory day-care centers. In either setting, however, the treatment requires an extended period away from the patient's normal activities. Thus, combining the high cost of hospitalization or day-care with the loss of income incurred by many people, this is an expensive approach to treatment, particularly when compared to other treatment modalities that provide similar results.

The Treatment is Messy and Malodorous

Psoriatic patients are already unhappy with their skin and application of crude coal tar all over their body smacks strongly of the "pain builds character" notion. Refined tars have been substituted for crude coal tar in some modifications of the Goeckerman treatment because they are more cosmetically acceptable. However, they appear to be less active than crude coal tar and in some instances have had all detectable therapeutic effect refined out of them.

The Treatment Lacks a Maintenance Component

The patient is usually cleared of disease but after discharge from treatment, psoriasis generally returns. Some authors refer to a 50% relapse rate at 1 year, a relapse meaning that the disease has returned to its original state. Since the return is gradual in most instances, this means that many of these patients would have had significant disease for most of the year.

Among physicians, there are still many strong supporters of the Goeckerman regimen who argue for its safety and efficacy. Besides, it does not require any understanding of complicated photobiology; it is just a comfortable treatment that almost always works. However, most patients do not share this comfortable feeling. The acid test is to talk to patients who have been treated with the Goeckerman regimen and also have been treated with UVB phototherapy or PUVA therapy; the Goeckerman regimen then has few supporters. However, we do not have to decide this issue since the federal government and third-party carriers are already deciding that prolonged hospitalization for psoriasis and use of day-care facilities are too expensive.

TAR PHOTOSENSITIZATION

Goeckerman originally intended to use tar photosensitization to treat psoriasis, which would have been an early version of photochemotherapy. However, although tar is phototoxic, its action spectrum is in the UVA waveband, and he was using a radiation source with a peak emission in the UVB waveband. Despite that initial error, tar photochemotherapy remained a potential therapeutic approach to psoriasis. The possibility has been explored in two ways and although neither is useful, they are worth mentioning.

In a bilateral comparison study of tar plus UVA radiation to one side of the body and tar plus UVB radiation to the other side, we found that both sides responded equally; equierythemogenic doses of both treatments were used. However, tar phototoxicity is associated with a "smarting" reaction in the skin. This phenomenon, previously described in pitch workers, consists of an unpleasant burning pain in exposed skin that begins at various intervals after commencing exposure to UVA radiation and subsides within seconds of stopping irradiation. All patients in our study experienced the reaction and at times it was severe enough to interrupt treatment. Therefore, tar photosensitization alone is not a practical approach to treatment. The cause of the smarting reaction is not known but presumably involves phototoxic injury to selected nerve fibers in the skin.

The second approach to using tar photosensitization therapeutically has been to modify the Goeckerman regimen by the addition of a small amount of this component. Thus, the therapeutic components of this regimen become tar, UVB, and tar photosensitization with UVA by the addition of a significant dose of UVA radiation. This is an interesting modification, but even when the dose of UVA radiation is raised to a "stinging" dose, it is not possible to detect a significant therapeutic effect from tar phototoxicity.

HOME PHOTOTHERAPY

Treatment using a UVB phototherapy unit installed at home appears at first glance to be a very attractive option but the pros and cons require careful consideration by both the physician and the patient.

The Treatment

Both narrowband and broadband UVB are available from several manufacturers and usually consist of one or two panels. Dosimetry is usually measured in minutes and the patient starts with a low dose and uses erythema as a guide to increments in the dose. Treatment frequency varies, but three to five treatments a week is usually advised. Combined treatment with tar and suberythemagenic doses of UVB radiation at home has also been reported as effective.

Advantages

Convenience and cost are usually cited as the main advantages of home phototherapy. Obviously, convenience is a large plus for the patients since they no longer have to come to the clinic for treatment. Some insurance companies will reimburse the patient for purchase of a unit and thus for the patient, the cost can be low.

Disadvantages

There are a number of potential problems that deter many physicians:

Physician Input

Home therapy requires considerable time and effort on the part of the physician. Patients must first be carefully screened for strong motivation and reliability to ensure good compliance and adequate follow-up. The patients must be fully instructed in how to perform the treatment and warned of all possible adverse effects. Arrangements must be made for obtaining or constructing a suitable radiator. The physician must be available for numerous telephone calls when the patient seeks further advice.

Lack of Follow-up

The patients are being provided with an "open prescription" for a potentially dangerous treatment, since there is no guarantee that they will return for follow-up evaluations. Even patients who appear to be reliable and intelligent can become lost to follow-up and continue to manage their own treatment for years. One phototherapy equipment company has attempted to avoid this problem by programming units to deliver a limited number of treatments. However, a handyman can easily circumvent this safeguard.

Lack of Control of Treatment

Home phototherapy by its very nature is poorly controlled, from the standpoint of both radiometry and dose. The physician who just advises his or her patients to buy a solarium will have no idea what radiation the patient is receiving. In the best of situations in which a specified lamp is used, there is usually no provision for regular monitoring of the irradiance of the system. This lack of control usually results in the patient's receiving much more treatment, to achieve any given end point, than would have been used in an office or clinic.

Legal Problems

The legal implications of advising a patient about home therapy with an indoor radiator are not clear. If the physician provides advice on the construction of such a unit, responsibility for its safe function may well rest with the physician.

Insurance Problems

If a patient has been reimbursed for purchase of a home unit but then finds it is not effective, some insurance companies will refuse to reimburse for subsequent clinic treatment.

Conclusions

Occasionally, the situation arises in which a patient who is well known to the physician cannot come for treatment in the clinic for geographic or social reasons. Consideration can then be given to home phototherapy. However, an entire program of home phototherapy for the treatment of psoriasis requires a large commitment of time and energy by the physician. It is not clear that this approach is preferable to clinic treatment for either patients or physicians.

CLIMATOTHERAPY

This term is used to include heliotherapy where sun is used as the source of UV radiation and balneophototherapy, in which exposure to the sun or an indoor source of UV is combined with bathing, usually in a salt solution. The Dead Sea in Israel has the most well-developed facilities for climatotherapy but other sites reporting this treatment are the Canary Islands, Yugoslavia, and Iceland. In addition, some clinics have attempted to replicate balneophototherapy using indoor bathing in Dead Sea salt solutions and exposure to narrowband UVB phototherapy.

The Treatment

At the Dead Sea, patients stay in hotels and spend most of their time in the treatment facility with a daily program of bathing, exposure to sunlight, and application of moisturizers and keratolytics. A typical stay is 4 weeks.

Mechanism of Treatment

There are several components to treatment at the Dead Sea and the contribution of each to the beneficial effect in psoriasis has not been determined.

Selective UV Phototherapy

This is probably the main factor in improving psoriasis. The Dead Sea is 390 m below sea level and therefore sunlight there passes through a greater thickness of atmosphere, which filters out the more erythemogenic wavelengths shorter than 300 nm. Consequently, patients can expose themselves to sunlight for long periods of time each day and receive very high doses of radiation of wavelengths longer than 300 nm, which is more therapeutic for psoriasis.

Psychotherapeutic Effects

Patients are on vacation and associate with other people with psoriasis and both these factors are probably important components of the treatment.

Supervised Topical Program

Regular application of topical medication such as tar and keratolytic agents, plus assisted treatment for scalp psoriasis, contributes to the overall therapy.

Bathing in a Salt Solution

Water in the Dead Sea contains salts, mainly magnesium and sodium chlorides, in a concentration of 30% as compared to 3% in seawater. Anecdotal claims of benefit from bathing in this salt solution are made but bilateral comparison studies indicate that bathing in water increases the effectiveness of phototherapy without any additional benefit from the salt. Regardless, the Dead Sea is a unique setting, so the claim of therapeutic benefit from its salts is at least good for advertising if not for psoriasis.

Advantages of the Treatment

Climatotherapy is effective with about 85% of patients cleared or markedly improved in 4 weeks. It is also probably fairly safe although one study found a significantly increased frequency of nonmelanoma skin in patients treated with climatotherapy; the role of the treatment in this finding could not be determined.

Disadvantages of the Treatment

There are two main drawbacks of climatotherapy.

Cost

Travel, hotel, and treatment costs make this a very expensive therapy as compared to conventional phototherapy. The added expense of being away from work for 4 weeks further contributes to the cost.

Lack of Maintenance

Obviously, there is no maintenance phase in most forms of climatotherapy, so many patients will relapse in a few months. Long remissions have been claimed but there is no evidence that they are longer than the remission following any other short-term course of phototherapy.

TANNING PARLOR PHOTOTHERAPY

A surprising number of dermatologists and their patients use tanning parlors for management of psoriasis. At first glance this seems quite logical: tanning beds emit UV radiation and UV radiation is therapeutic in psoriasis.

The Treatment

Most tanning parlors use fluorescent bulbs that emit mostly UVA radiation because this wavelength is most effective for producing a tan. The protocol used is dictated by the operator of the tanning parlor whose aim is to tan the individual and lacks any knowledge about treatment of psoriasis.

Advantages

Cost and convenience are the two main advantages suggested by physicians and patients using this treatment. In addition, most patients do achieve some improvement in their psoriasis probably due to the small amount of UVB emitted by the lamps.

Disadvantages

Few patients ever clear their psoriasis and many reach a state of being deeply tanned with psoriasis still very evident. The reason is simple. Excessive melanogenesis is induced in both normal skin and the plaques of psoriasis so that therapeutic radiation can no longer reach its target in the dermis.

BIBLIOGRAPHY

Goeckerman Regimen

Le Vine MJ, White HAD, Parrish JA. Components of the Goeckerman regimen. J Invest Dermatol 1979; 73:170–173.

Perry HO, Soderstrom CW, Schulze RW. The Goeckerman treatment of psoriasis. Arch Dermatol 1968; 98:178–182.

Stern RS, Gange RW, Parrish JA, Tang SV, Arndt KA. Contribution of topical tar oil to ultraviolet B phototherapy for psoriasis. J Am Acad Dermatol 1986; 14:742–747.

Tannenbaum L, Parrish JA, Pathak MA, Anderson RR, Fitzpatrick TB. Tar phototoxicity and phototherapy for psoriasis. Arch Dermatol 1975; 111:467–470.

Tar Photosensitization

Diette KM, Gange RW, Stern RS, Arndt KA, Parrish JA. Coal tar phototoxicity: characteristics of the smarting reaction. J Invest Dermatol 1985; 84:268–271.

Parrish JA, Morison WL, Gonzalez E, Krop TM, White HAD, Rosario R. Therapy of psoriasis by tar photosensitization. J Invest Dermatol 1978; 70:111–112.

Home Phototherapy

Feldman SR, Clark A, Reboussin DM, Fleischer AB. An assessment of potential problems of home phototherapy treatment of psoriasis. Cutis 1996; 58:71–73.

Larkö O, Swanbeck G. Home solarium treatment of psoriasis. Br J Dermatol 1979; 101:13–16.

Sarkany RPE, Anstey A, Diffey BL, Jobling R, Langmack K, McGregor JM, Moseley H, Murphy GM, Rhodes LE, Norris PG. Home phototherapy: report on a workshop of the British Photodermatology Group, December 1996. Br J Dermatol 1999; 140:195–199.

Climatotherapy

Abels DJ, Kattan-Byron J. Psoriasis treatment at the Dead Sea: a natural selective ultraviolet phototherapy. J Am Acad Dermatol 1985; 12:639–643.

Azizi E, Kushelevsky AP, Avrach W, Schewach-Millet M. Climate therapy for psoriasis at the Dead Sea, Israel. Isr J Med Sci 1982; 18:267–270.

Frentz G, Olsen JH, Avrach WW. Malignant tumours and psoriasis: climatotherapy at the Dead Sea. Br J Dermatol 1999; 141:1088–1091.

Gambichler T, Rapp S, Senger E, Altmeyer P, Hoffman K. Balneophother-
apy of psoriasis: highly concentrated salt water versus tap
water—a randomized, one-blind, right/left comparative study. Photodermatol Photoimmunol Photomed 2001; 17:22–25.

Halevy S, Sukenik S. Different modalities of spa therapy for skin diseases at
the Dead Sea area. Arch Dermatol 1998; 134:1416–1420.

Kushelevsky AP, Harari M, Kudish AI, Hristakieva E, Ingber A, Shani J.
Safety of solar phototherapy at the Dead Sea. J Am Acad Dermatol
1998; 38:447–452.

Molin L. Climate therapy for Swedish psoriatics on Hvar, Yugoslavia. Acta
Derm Venereol (Stockh) 1972; 52:155–160.

Mork C, Wahl A. Improved quality of life among patients with psoriasis
after supervised climate therapy at the Canary Islands. J Am Acad
Dermatol 2002; 47:314–316.

Ólafsson JH, Sigurgeirsson B, Pálsdóttir R. Psoriasis treatment: bathing in a
thermal lagoon combined with UVB, versus UVB treatment only.
Acta Derm Venereol (Stockh) 1996; 76:228–230.

Snellman E. Comparison of the antipsoriatic efficacy of heliotherapy and
ultraviolet B: a cross-over study. Photodermatol Photoimmunol
Photomed 1992; 9:83–85.

Snellman E, Maljanen T, Aromaa A, Reunanen A, Jyrkinen-
Pakkasvirta T, Luoma J. Effect of heliotherapy on the cost of psoriasis. Br J Dermatol 1998; 138:288–;292.

Tanning Parlor Phototherapy

Carlin CS, Callis KP, Krueger GG. Efficacy of acitretin and commercial
tanning bed therapy for psoriasis. Arch Dermatol 2003; 139:436–442.

Das S, Lloyd JJ, Walshaw D, Diffey BL, Farr PM. Response of psoriasis to
sunbed treatment: comparison of conventional ultraviolet A lamps
with new higher ultraviolet B-emitting lamps. Br J Dermatol 2002;
147:966–972.

Ferguson J. A controlled study of ultraviolet A sunbed treatment of
psoriasis. Br J Dermatol 2000; 143:919–922.

Parrish JA. Treatment of psoriasis with long-wave ultraviolet light. Arch
Dermatol 1977; 113:1525–1528.

Turner RJ, Walshaw D, Diffey BL, Farr PM. A controlled study of ultraviolet A sunbed treatment of psoriasis. Br J Dermatol 2000; 143:
957–963.

13

Combination Therapy

INTRODUCTION

Every agent known to have an antipsoriatic effect has been used in combination with UV therapy and some have been fairly thoroughly evaluated. An important question to consider before using a combination therapy is: has the combination treatment been shown to be more effective than the primary treatment used alone? At first glance this question might sound silly and evoke a response of two agents must be better than one, but this is not necessarily true. Tar clearly is effective in psoriasis but, as discussed earlier, when combined with erythemogenic doses of UVB radiation no therapeutic effect of tar can be detected. Or put more simply, the weak therapeutic effect of tar is swamped by the more potent therapeutic activity of UVB radiation. Therefore, it is important to establish the therapeutic benefit of a second agent; otherwise the patient could be exposed to unnecessary potential adverse effects from that agent.

There are two reasons for using a second or even a third agent in combination with UV therapy: to improve efficacy and to reduce long-term adverse effects of exposure to UV radiation. According to this reasoning, combination treatment would be used in all patients, but in reality it is mainly used to improve efficacy when it is considered that UV therapy alone will not be sufficient to clear disease. The specific indications for when combination must be considered are listed in Table 1. The last of those indications applies to the commercial salesperson who is seldom in town, the

Table 1   Specific Indications for Combination Therapy

Skin type IV–VI
Asbestos and coral-plaque disease
Previous failed or partial response to UV therapy
Extensive inflammatory psoriasis
Social or geographic problems requiring rapid clearance

---

globe-trotting executive, and the patient who lives 50 mi away, all of whom
are candidates for a short intensive course of therapy.

PUVA/BROADBAND UVB THERAPY

This is the simplest combination treatment since it does not require a
detailed explanation to the patient. There are two situations in which it
can be used.

Initial Clearance Therapy

Both treatments are commenced simultaneously at the initiation of therapy
and if a combination unit is available, both treatments can be given at the
same time (Table 2). In bilateral comparison studies, this regimen resulted
in a marked reduction in cumulative exposure to both UVA and UVB radiation, and more rapid clearance of psoriasis as compared to PUVA therapy
alone. This combined treatment should be considered for all skin type
IV–VI patients.

Add-on Therapy

When a patient is showing a slow response during a course of PUVA therapy and has developed marked pigmentation or has reached the dose of
UVA radiation suitable for his or her skin type, addition of broadband
UVB radiation may provide the boost necessary to clear (Table 3). The
initial dose of UVB can be determined by doing an MED or on the basis
of skin type.

Table 2   PUVA/UVB as Initial Clearance Therapy

T.I.W. or 11011 treatment
Regular PUVA schedule
High-dose broadband UVB schedule
Both treatments given at the same time
Maintenance: PUVA alone or PUVA/UVB

Table 3 PUVA/UVB as an Add-on Therapy

Problem is pigmentation: increase UVA dose
Problem is a high dose of UVA: hold UVA dose
Start UVB at 70% MED
Or, if skin type
  I: $60\,mJ/cm^2$
  II: $100\,mJ/cm^2$
  III: $140\,mJ/cm^2$
  IV: $180\,mJ/cm^2$
  V: $240\,mJ/cm^2$
  VI: $300\,mJ/cm^2$
Increase dose of UVB by 20% each treatment

What is the Cause of Erythema?

The good news is that erythema is not more common using a PUVA/UVB combined therapy but since an erythemogenic schedule for broadband UVB therapy is being used, erythemas will occur. It is necessary to determine which waveband is the cause. This is simply done by history since erythema starting a few hours after treatment is due to UVB, while if it is delayed in onset to 36 hr or more after treatment, it is due to PUVA.

Maintenance Therapy

When the patient has been cleared on a combination PUVA and UVB schedule, UVB therapy is usually stopped and maintenance treatment consists of PUVA therapy alone. The main reason for stopping UVB phototherapy is the problem of erythema from this waveband when it is used as a maintenance treatment. However, in some situations maintenance therapy with both wavebands must be given. The main indications for this are very active and aggressive disease and a high skin type. In these cases, the frequency of maintenance will usually have to be held at weekly or every other week treatment.

Two Caveats

First, when using PUVA/UVB therapy as a clearance treatment, the frequency of treatment has to be at least T.I.W. since in a B.I.W. schedule over half the patients gain no advantage over PUVA therapy alone. Second, narrowband UVB cannot be substituted for broadband UVB radiation unless the physician is planning on developing a new treatment schedule. The reason is simple: narrowband UVB activates psoralen and broadband UVB radiation does not. So if narrowband UVB radiation is used in combination with PUVA therapy the patient is being treated with PUVA plus psoralen/narrowband UVB and narrowband UVB radiation and this treatment schedule has not been explored.

ACITRETIN

Short-Term Therapy

A combination treatment using UV therapy as the primary treatment and acitretin, a retinoid marketed under the trade name of Soriatane®, has been used as a clearance treatment for psoriasis, particularly in Europe. Prior to approval of acitretin, the precursor etretinate was used in many early studies. Acitretin has been combined with narrowband UVB therapy, broadband UVB therapy, and PUVA therapy. The combined therapy is used with the aims of reducing the number of treatments to clear disease, reducing the total cumulative dose of UV radiation, and increasing the percentage of patients having a successful response to treatment. Some studies have reported success in achieving all these aims, some have partially achieved them, and others have reported negative results. Analysis of the methods and results of these studies suggests that this combined treatment is useful provided two criteria are met:

- Acitretin should be given in a dose of 1 mg/kg body weight; lower doses are not beneficial.
- Acitretin should be commenced 10–14 days before UV therapy is started.

Acitretin and UV therapy are continued together until the disease is controlled, at which stage acitretin is stopped and the patient is maintained on UV therapy alone.

Long-Term Therapy

There have been suggestions that acitretin be used in a low dose (25 mg daily) on a long-term basis in combination with UV therapy, particularly PUVA therapy, to reduce the carcinogenic potential of these treatments. There are no prospective studies to support this idea but it may have value, particularly in patients at high risk of developing skin cancer.

Contraindications

Acitretin should not be used in women of child-bearing potential. It is markedly teratogenic and contraception is required for 3 years after cessation of the drug and no one can guarantee such compliance. It is also relatively contraindicated in patients with hyperlipidemia unless this is corrected, and in patients with evidence of liver disease.

Monitoring

Serum lipids and liver function tests are necessary before starting therapy, 2 weeks into treatment and then monthly.

Adverse Effects

The major adverse effects are hyperlipidemia and abnormal liver function. Minor mucucutaneous, "nuisance" side effects, occur in most patients even in low-dose treatment. These include cheilitis, sticky skin and dryness, and irritation of the eyes. Increased photosensitivity has been mentioned by some authors as a problem when using acitretin in combination with UV therapy, but in practice this has not been evident.

METHOTREXATE

Short-Term Therapy

Methotrexate has been used as a clearance treatment in combination with broadband UVB therapy and PUVA therapy with a reduction in the number of exposures to UV and the total dose of UV radiation. The combination of narrowband UVB therapy and methotrexate has not been evaluated in a study but appears to give similar results in practice. The schedule for PUVA/methotrexate is outlined in Table 4. Rebound of psoriasis after methotrexate is stopped can be a problem but this appears to occur only in patients with very high inflammatory disease and in patients kept on methotrexate for more than 2 months. In both instances, the rebound can usually be controlled by a return to a clearance course of UV therapy.

Contraindications

Methotrexate is highly teratogenic and women of child-bearing potential must use contraception while on the medication and for a month after it is stopped. Advanced liver and renal diseases are contraindications to using methotrexate. Abnormal liver function tests are not a contraindication for a short course of treatment, but they should be monitored weekly. In patients with moderate impairment of renal function and any patient over 70 years of age, the dose of methotrexate should be halved.

Monitoring

A blood count and metabolic panel should be obtained at baseline, a test dose of 5 mg methotrexate is given, the blood count is repeated 5 days later, and then repeat tests at 2-week intervals.

Table 4 Combination PUVA/methotrexate therapy

Methotrexate 5 mg Q 12 hr × 3 doses QW for 3 weeks
Then start PUVA therapy T.I.W. or 11011 and continue methotrexate
At clearance, stop methotrexate and start maintenance PUVA therapy

---

Adverse Effects

Bone marrow suppression is the main adverse effect of methotrexate therapy when given as a short course of treatment but fortunately this is rare and should be detected by blood tests. Unexpected erythemal reactions were common in the original study of this combined treatment, but fortunately, this has not continued to be a problem.

CYCLOSPORIN

Combining cyclosporin with UV therapy would appear to be contraindicated in all but the most extreme circumstances because of the increased risk of skin cancer when using this immunosuppressive agent. In addition, in one study evaluating this combination more than half the patients had a severe relapse during the 6 months following clearance.

TOPICAL AGENTS

The various topical antipsoriatic agents have all been used in combination with each UV therapy and in general they accelerate clearance of psoriasis. However, in practice these agents are mainly used as adjunctive treatment to augment therapy of plaques that are slow to respond such as on the knees, elbows, and lower legs. There is a very practical reason why topical agents are not used over extensive areas as a combination treatment with UV therapy: the patients do not like the idea. By the time they start UV therapy they have already used topical therapies without a satisfactory response and they want to stop this losing approach to treatment.

Calcipotriene

This agent is usually well tolerated during UV therapy and aids clearance of resistant plaques. A few cases of temporary hyperpigmentation at sites of plaques treated with PUVA plus calcipotriene have been reported but this does not appear to be a common event. A thick layer applied immediately before exposure to UV radiation can act as a sunscreen and the calcipotriene is inactivated by UVA radiation. Therefore, patients should be warned to apply calcipotriene several hours before exposure or only after exposure to UV therapy.

Topical Corticosteroids

These agents are also useful in helping clear resistant areas of disease and are usually well tolerated. Extensive use of high-potency steroids or use of these agents with occlusion may destabilize psoriasis and lead to relapses during maintenance treatment.

Tazarotene

This agent is frequently associated with irritation of the skin and has poor patient acceptability. It probably also causes photosensitivity due to thinning of the skin so it should be used with caution in combination with UV therapy.

BIOLOGIC THERAPIES

When we gain more experience using the newer systemic agents, termed biologic therapy, for treatment of psoriasis they will certainly be used in combination with UV therapy. The combined treatments will likely be superior to either agent used as monotherapy, but the larger question of what the safety profile is for such a combination will take years to answer. The claim is that these biologic agents are selective, targeted treatments, but they do have profound effects on the immune system. What effect they will have on the incidence of skin cancer is an important question.

WHY IS COMBINATION THERAPY NOT ROUTINE?

Only a minority of physicians appear to use combination therapies and even then only in a minority of their patients. The main reason why combination therapy is not used more frequently is the complexity of the undertaking. Introducing a new patient to UV therapy, particularly PUVA therapy, is complex by itself since apart from the evaluation, the therapy, its potential adverse effect, and precautions to be taken, all have to be explained. To introduce the patient to a second treatment such as acitretin or methotrexate at the same time can be overwhelming for both the physician and the patient. However, consideration should be given to combination therapy the second time around when the patient is already familiar with UV therapy and the physician/patient relationship is established.

BIBLIOGRAPHY

Reviews

Fritsch P, Hönigsmann H. Combination phototherapy—a critical appraisal. Curr Probl Dermatol 1986; 15:238–253.

Lebwohl M, Menter A, Koo J, Feldman SR. Combination therapy to treat moderate to severe psoriasis. J Am Acad Dermatol 2004; 50:416–430.

Morison WL. PUVA combination therapy. Photodermatology 1985; 2:229–236.

Weinstein GD, White GM. An approach to the treatment of moderate to severe psoriasis with rotational therapy. J Am Acad Dermatol 1993; 28:454–459.

PUVA/UVB Therapy

Diette KM, Momtaz-T K, Stern RS, Arndt KA, Parrish JA. Psoralens and UV-A and UV-B twice weekly for the treatment of psoriasis. Arch Dermatol 1984; 120:1169–1173.

Momtaz TK, Parrish JA. Combination of psoralens and ultraviolet A and ultraviolet B in the treatment of psoriasis vulgaris: a bilateral comparison study. J Am Acad Dermatol 1984; 10:481–486.

Morison WL. Combination of methoxsalen and ultraviolet B (UVB) vs. UVB radiation alone in treatment of psoriasis: a bilateral comparison study. Photodermatol Photoimmunol Photomed 1995; 11:6–8.

Ortel B, Perl S, Kinaciyan T, Calzavara-Pinton PG, Hönigsmann H. Comparison of narrow-band (311 nm) UVB and broad-band UVA after oral or bath-water 8-methoxypsoralen in the treatment of psoriasis. J Am Acad Dermatol 1993; 29:736–740.

Sakuntabhai A, Diffey BL, Farr PM. Response of psoriasis to psoralen-UVB photochemotherapy. Br J Dermatol 1993; 128:296–300.

Retinoids

Fritsch PO, Hönigsman H, Jaschke E, Wolff K. Augmentation of oral methoxsalen-photochemotherapy with an oral retinoic acid derivative. J Invest Dermatol 1978; 70:178–182.

Green C, Lakshmipathi T, Johnson BE, Ferguson J. A comparison of the efficacy and relapse rates of narrowband UVB (TL-01) monotherapy vs. etretinate (re-TL-01) vs. etretinate-PUVA (re-PUVA) in the treatment of psoriasis patients. Br J Dermatol 1992; 127:5–9.

Hudson-Peacock MJ, Angus B, Farr PM. Response of PUVA-induced keratoses to etretinate. J Am Acad Dermatol 1996; 35:120–123.

Lebwohl M, Drake L, Menter A, Koo J, Gottlieb AB, Zanolli M, Young M, McClelland P. Consensus conference: acitretin in combination with UVB or PUVA in the treatment of psoriasis. J Am Acad Dermatol 2001; 45:544–553.

Lowe NJ, Prystowsky JH, Bourget T, Edelstein J, Nychay S, Armstrong R. Acitretin plus UVB therapy for psoriasis. J Am Acad Dermatol 1991; 24:591–594.

Nijsten TEC, Stern TS. Oral retinoid use reduces cutaneous squamous cell carcinoma risk in patients with psoriasis treated with psoralen-UVA: a nested cohort study. J Am Acad Dermatol 2003; 49:644–650.

Orfanos CE, Steigleder GK, Pullmann H, Bloch PH. Oral retinoid and UVB radiation: a new, alternative treatment for psoriasis on an out-patient basis. Acta Dermatol 1979; 59:241–244.

Parker S, Coburn P, Lawrence C, Marks J, Shuster S. A randomized double-blind comparison of PUVA-etretinate and PUVA-placebo in the treatment of chronic plaque psoriasis. Br J Dermatol 1984; 110:215–220.

Ruzicka T, Sommerburg C, Braun-Falco O, Mult HC, Köster W, Lengen W, Lensing W, Letzel H, Meigel WN, Paul E, Przybilla B, Steinert M, Winzer M, Wiskemann A. Efficiency of acitretin in combination with UV-B in the treatment of severe psoriasis. Arch Dermatol 1990; 126:482–486.

Tanew A, Guggenbichler A, Hönigsmann H, Geiger JM, Fritsch P. Photochemotherapy for severe psoriasis without or in combination with acitretin: a randomized, double-blind comparison study. J Am Acad Dermatol 1991; 25:682–684.

Saurat JH, Geiger JM, Amblard P, Beani JC, Boulanger A, Claudy A, Frenk E, Guilhou JJ, Grosshans E, Mérot Y, Meynadier J, Tapernoux B. Randomized double-blind multicenter study comparison acitretin-PUVA, etretinate-PUVA and placebo-PUVA in the treatment of severe psoriasis. Dermatologica 1988; 177:218–224.

Methotrexate

Morison WL, Momtaz K, Parrish JA, Fitzpatrick TB. Combined methotrexate-PUVA therapy in the treatment of psoriasis. J Am Acad Dermatol 1982; 6:46–51.

Paul BS, Momtaz TK, Stern RS, Arndt KA, Parrish JA. Combined methotrexate-ultraviolet B therapy in the treatment of psoriasis. J Am Acad Dermatol 1982; 7:758–762.

Cyclosporin

Petzelbauer P, Hönigsmann H, Langer K, Anegg B, Strohal R, Tanew A, Wolff K. Cyclosporin A in combination with photochemotherapy (PUVA) in the treatment of psoriasis. Br J Dermatol 1990; 123:641–647.

Calcipotriene

Brands S, Brakman M, Bos JD, de Rie MA. No additional effect of calcipotriol ointment on low-dose narrow-band UVB phototherapy in psoriasis. J Am Acad Dermatol 1999; 41:991–995.

Gläser R, Röwert J, Mrowietz U. Hyperpigmentation due to topical calcipotriol and photochemotherapy in two psoriatic patients. Br J Dermatol 1998; 139:148–151.

Kokelj F, Plozzir C. Reduction of UV-A radiation induced by calcipotriol in the treatment of vulgar psoriasis with oral psoralen plus UV-A. Arch Dermatol 1997; 133:668–669.

Kerscher M, Volkenandt M, Plewig G, Lehmann P. Combination phototherapy of psoriasis with calcipotriol and narrow-band UVB. Lancet 1993; 342:923.

Kragballe K. Combination of topical calcipotriol (MC 903) and UVB radiation for psoriasis vulgaris. Dermatologica 1990; 181:211–214.

Lehmann P, Kerscher M. Combination phototherapy of psoriasis with calcipotriene and narrow-band (311 nm) UVB. J Am Acad Dermatol 1997; 36:501.

McKenna KE, Stern RS. Photosensitivity associated with combined UV-B and calcipotriene therapy. Arch Dermatol 1995; 131:1305–1307.

Rim JH, Choe YB, Youn JI. Positive effect of using calcipotriol ointment with narrow-band ultraviolet B phototherapy in psoriatic patients. Photodermatol Photoimmunol Photomed 2002; 18:131–134.

Speight EL, Farr PM. Calcipotriol improves the response of psoriasis to PUVA. Br J Dermatol 1994; 130:79–82.

Woo WK, McKenna KE. Combination TL01 ultraviolet B phototherapy and topical calcipotriol for psoriasis: a prospective randomized placebo-controlled clinical trial. Br J Dermatol 2003; 149:146–150.

Corticosteroids

Dover JS, McEvoy MT, Rosen CF, Arndt KA, Stern RS. Are topical corticosteroids useful in phototherapy for psoriasis? J Am Acad Dermatol 1989; 20:748–754.

Larkö O, Swanbeck G, Svartholm H. The effect on psoriasis of clobetasol propionate used alone or in combination with UVB. Acta Dermatol Venereol 1984; 64:151–154.

LeVine MJ, Parrish JA. The effect of topical fluocinonide ointment on phototherapy of psoriasis. J Invest Dermatol 1982; 78:157–159.

Morison WL, Parrish JA, Fitzpatrick TB. Controlled study of PUVA and adjunctive topical therapy in the management of psoriasis. Br J Dermatol 1978; 98:125–132.

Petrozzi JW. Topical steroids and UV radiation in psoriasis. Arch Dermatol 1983; 119:207–210.

Tazarotene

Behrens S, Grundmann-Kollmann M, Schiener R, Peter RU, Kerscher M. Combination phototherapy of psoriasis with narrow-band UVB irradiation and topical tazarotene gel. J Am Acad Dermatol 2000; 42:493–495.

Hecker D, Worsley J, Yueh G, Kuroda K, Lebwohl M. Interactions between tazarotene and ultraviolet light. J Am Acad Dermatol 1999; 41:927–930.

Koo JYM, Lowe NJ, Lew-Kaya DA, Vasilopoulos AI, Lue JC, Sefton J, Gibson JR. Tazarotene plus UVB phototherapy in the treatment of psoriasis. J Am Acad Dermatol 2000; 43:821–828.

Schiener R, Behrens-Williams SC, Pillekamp H, Kaskel P, Peter RU, Kerscher M. Calcipotriol vs. tazarotene as combination therapy with narrowband ultraviolet B (311 nm): efficacy in patients with severe psoriasis. Br J Dermatol 2000; 143:1275–1278.

Tzaneve S, Seeber A, Hönigsmann H, Tanew A. A comparison of psoralen plus ultraviolet A (PUVA) monotherapy, tacalcitol plus PUVA and tazarotene plus PUVA in patients with chronic plaque-type psoriasis. Br J Dermatol 2002; 147:748–753.

Treatment of Other Diseases

Once PUVA therapy was found to be an effective treatment for psoriasis vulgaris, considerable interest was focused on its efficacy in other diseases so that the therapeutic spectrum of the treatment has broadened and is still being defined. In contrast, interest in UVB phototherapy has mainly centered on plaque-type psoriasis, although this is beginning to change with wider use of narrowband therapy.

Part of the motivation for trying UV radiation therapy in various diseases can be attributed to a "let us try it and see what happens" attitude, and this particularly applies to diseases for which there is no effective treatment. However, this is changing to a more scientifically sound motivation based on the supposed mechanism of action of the treatments. The finding that UV therapy of psoriasis results in elimination of activated T lymphocytes from the skin is consistent with the theory of selective cytotoxicity as a mechanism of action. According to this concept the treatments work via selective killing of a cell or cells in the skin that are responsible for mediating the disease in question. In support of this hypothesis is the observation that all diseases that have responded to the treatments are characterized by the presence of inflammatory cells or other abnormal accumulations of cells, and when tested, these cells are very sensitive to photons.

14

Psoriasis Variants

INTRODUCTION

Despite a fairly uniform response of psoriasis vulgaris to PUVA and UVB phototherapy, the results achieved in other forms of the disease and its near relatives have been more mixed. This is partly due to the nature of the disease and partly to the photobiological limitations of the treatments. In general, combination treatment with addition of a retinoid or methotrexate is more often indicated under these conditions.

GENERALIZED PUSTULAR PSORIASIS

Nature of Disease

The generalized form of pustular psoriasis, named after the original case reported by von Zumbusch, can arise spontaneously in a patient with psoriasis vulgaris or be triggered by some event. Withdrawal of systemic corticosteroids used for treatment of psoriasis or some other concurrent disease is the most common trigger and withdrawal of intensive topical therapy with a potent corticosteroid, such as clobetasol propionate, can have a similar effect. Pregnancy and infection are other triggers.

The severity of the disease varies greatly. In its milder form the patient has extensive, painful, inflammatory psoriasis with scattered pustules, no systemic symptoms, and a moderate leucocytosis. The severe form of the disease can be life-threatening with extensive erythema covered with pustules, high fever, malaise, and a marked leucocytosis.

Management

Severe cases of generalized pustular psoriasis should be hospitalized, while moderate cases can be treated on an ambulatory basis. The management is outlined in Table 1.

Suppress Inflammation

The choice of the agent for control of inflammation depends on the individual circumstances of the patient and the severity of the disease. Acitretin, in a dose of 1 mg/kg body weight daily, is the agent of choice since it controls pustulation within days. If this is contraindicated, as in women of child-bearing age, or in a patient with raised serum lipids, methotrexate (5 mg × 3 doses at 12 hr intervals each week) is an alternative in moderate cases but it usually takes several weeks to suppress pustulation. In severely ill patients systemic corticosteroids may be considered since they will rapidly suppress inflammation albeit with a significant price of complicating an already complicated situation. When the steroids are withdrawn, another systemic agent will have to be used to prevent a rebound of pustular psoriasis. Finally, cyclosporin should be considered as it also provides rapid control of disease but again, the disease will return once this agent is stopped. Cyclosporin does have the advantage that it can be used in pregnancy in extreme situations.

Control of Psoriasis

After 2 to 3 weeks of acitretin or 4 weeks of methotrexate, the inflammation is usually suppressed sufficiently to allow introduction of some form of UV therapy. PUVA therapy is the treatment of choice in most patients since maintenance treatment is often required for a year or more. It is started

Table 1 Management of Generalized Pustular Psoriasis

Consider hospitalization
Suppress inflammation
  Acitretin, methotrexate
  Corticosteroids, cyclosporin
Supportive measures
  Treat infection
  Maintain hydration
  Pain relief
  Topical steroids and oatmeal baths
Control psoriasis
  PUVA or UVB therapy

---

as a clearance schedule (TIW, BIW, or 11011) while the acitretin or methotrexate is continued. When the patient is clear, the systemic agent can be stopped and a maintenance schedule of PUVA therapy commenced. In patients with high skin types, PUVA plus UVB therapy would be preferred and in children narrowband UVB phototherapy should be considered as an alternative option.

UV therapy alone is not sufficient to control some patients after an episode of pustular psoriasis and then consideration has to be given to using long-term combination therapy with a low dose of acitretin, methotrexate, or a biologic agent.

ERYTHRODERMIC PSORIASIS

Nature of Disease

Erythrodermic psoriasis may develop gradually from psoriasis vulgaris and be chronic or it may develop acutely, often precipitated by the same events that cause generalized pustular psoriasis. An acute onset of erythroderma may present a diagnostic problem to distinguish from other causes of an erythroderm unless there are other manifestations of psoriasis or a past history of typical disease.

Management

Erythrodermic psoriasis is very incapacitating but its management does not present the same emergency situation as with pustular psoriasis except in the rare instance of a sudden onset with lots of inflammation. Management is outlined in Table 2.

Suppress Inflammation

Acitretin is the agent of choice but methotrexate and cyclosporin may be considered depending on the presence of any contraindications to the use

Table 2 Management of Erythrodermic Psoriasis

Diagnosis to establish psoriasis as cause
Suppress inflammation
   Acitretin
   Methotrexate
   Cyclosporin
Supportive measures
   Maintain nutrition and hydration
   Topical steroids and oatmeal baths
Control psoriasis
   PUVA or UVB therapy

of a particular agent. The aim is to reduce the intensity of erythema as much as possible, and regain some skin with a normal appearance as a guide for UV therapy. This will take 2–3 weeks with acitretin or cyclosporin and about 4 weeks with methotrexate.

Control Psoriasis

The systemic agent is continued when UV therapy is commenced and the combination therapy is used until psoriasis is clear; the systemic agent is then stopped and maintenance UV therapy is continued. PUVA therapy is usually the treatment of choice since maintenance is often required for a year or more. PUVA plus UVB phototherapy should be considered in higher skin type individuals and narrowband UVB therapy may be considered in children.

There are two main problems during the clearance phase of treatment: recurrent phototoxicity and the diagnostic distinction between this adverse effect and the underlying disease. Patients with erythrodermic psoriasis should be treated with PUVA as if they were skin type I with low doses of UVA radiation and a nonaggressive approach to increases in the radiation dose. Redness from phototoxicity is difficult to distinguish from redness of the disease. Usually the only clues to the presence of clinical phototoxicity are complaints of pain and tenderness of the skin, and these symptoms are maximal in exposed areas. If there is doubt about the correct diagnosis, a bilateral comparison is often useful; treatment is continued on one half of the body and stopped on the other half. Usually, the responses on the two sides will differ after a few treatments. Because of these difficulties with treatment, attempts to clear erythrodermic psoriasis using UV therapy alone are seldom successful and such an approach is not advised.

Maintenance treatment is always required and should be tapered slowly over several months. In some patients, UV therapy is not sufficient to control disease and combination treatment with a low dose of methotrexate, acitretin, or a biologic agent must be used.

GUTTATE PSORIASIS

Nature of the Disease

Guttate psoriasis is usually of sudden onset developing over days to a week or more and it may appear in the absence of any previous evidence of psoriasis or may occur in a person with existing psoriasis. It is most common in younger patients and sometimes it can be recurrent over a period of years. The classic cause is an acute streptococcal throat infection and guttate psoriasis appears 10–14 days after symptoms of the infection begin. These days, nonspecific viral throat infections or infections of the urinary tract or elsewhere seem to be the triggers in many cases. A small proportion of patients with guttate psoriasis will undergo spontaneous remission and this can start as soon as 2 or 3 weeks after onset of the rash. However, most patients with guttate psoriasis if left untreated will evolve into chronic psoriasis and this has obvious implications for management.

Management

There are two goals of management: to avoid irritating the skin and to avoid leaving a patient with chronic psoriasis. Guttate psoriasis is a very unstable form of psoriasis and if the skin is irritated by treatment it may Koebnerize and become erythrodermic psoriasis. Irritants to be avoided include widespread UV-induced erythema, tar, and anthralin. Management is outlined in Table 3.

Diagnose and Treat Infection

The infection triggering the guttate psoriasis should be identified and treated when possible. Recurrent episodes of acute streptococcal throat infection may point to a need for tonsillectomy. However, there is no evidence that treatment of the underlying infection alters the course of guttate psoriasis.

Control of Psoriasis

Narrowband UVB phototherapy is the treatment of choice for skin types I–III and PUVA therapy is best for skin types IV–VI. Due to the lack of normal skin, phototesting is not an option, so conservative doses according to skin type should be used with the aim of avoiding erythema; after 6–10 treatments, psoriasis is usually suppressed sufficiently and erythema is no longer a concern.

Patients should be treated as soon as the diagnosis is made because the disease is the most responsive at that time and there is least risk of evolving into chronic psoriasis. In patients with no existing chronic psoriasis the goal is total clearance and this is usually achieved in 20–25 treatments and maintenance treatment is not required. Patients who had chronic psoriasis before the guttate episode require maintenance for a few months to ensure a remission.

Table 3 Management of Guttate Psoriasis

Diagnose and treat the infection
Narrowband UVB phototherapy or PUVA therapy
Cardinal rules
Treat early
Clear completely
Do not irritate the skin

PSORIASIS OF THE PALMS AND SOLES

Nature of the Disease

Psoriasis may be confined to the palms and soles resulting in significant morbidity by interfering with social interactions, and causing pain and discomfort during everyday activities. There are three main types of the disease, which may occur alone in a given patient or in various combinations in the same patient.

Psoriasis Vulgaris

Typical plaques of psoriasis may be confined to the palms and soles, although this variant is most common on the palms only.

Pustular Psoriasis

This is the commonest type of psoriasis on the palms and soles and includes many cases labeled as palmar-plantar pustulosis, which is probably a variant of psoriasis. Acrodermatitis continua of Hallopeau is a rare but distinctive variety of this disease.

Hyperkeratotic Psoriasis

Thick plaques are quite common and sometimes are so thick and devoid of obvious inflammation that they are mistakenly diagnosed as keratoderma.

It is important to define the type present in a given patient since the approach to treatment can vary with the type of the disease. In addition, there are patients who appear to have a crossover disease between psoriasis and eczema and these patients should be identified since their prognosis and treatment will be different if the true diagnosis is eczema.

Management

UV therapy can achieve clearance rates close to 100% with psoriasis on the palms and soles but this statement comes with some provisos. Psoriasis on the palms is more resistant to treatment compared to the disease elsewhere and the disease on the soles is more resistant than the disease on the palms. The problem is optical: how to get enough photons through the epidermis to suppress disease. For the same reason PUVA therapy is usually required to clear palms and soles and narrowband UVB therapy is usually not effective except in young children with thin disease.

Combination Therapy

A preliminary course of 3–4 weeks of acitretin (1 mg/kg body weight per day) or methotrexate (5 mg at 12 hr intervals for three doses weekly) before commencing UV therapy is the best approach to palm and sole psoriasis. This is mandatory with the hyperkeratotic form, desirable with the pustular form, and helpful with the plaque form. If systemic agents are contraindicated, attempts can be made to reduce hyperkeratosis with keratolytic agents such as Keralyt gel® under occlusion at night and to reduce inflammation with potent corticosteroids. However, successful clearance is much less likely to be achieved as compared with use of a systemic agent.

Oral PUVA Therapy

Oral administration of methoxsalen and exposure to UVA radiation in a manner similar to the treatment of psoriasis vulgaris elsewhere is my preferred approach to treatment. A radiator, specifically designed for treatment of the hands and feet, gives the best results, but an adequate result can be obtained with the door of a stand-up unit. A T.I.W. or 11011 schedule is a suitable protocol. The soles are slow to respond, presumably due to the thickness of the stratum corneum at that site, and increments of 1.0–1.5 J/cm^2 of UVA radiation should be used. Complete clearance is not always achieved or even desired by the patient. A remission of symptoms, particularly with disease on the soles, results in a very happy patient. The number of treatments required to produce a remission is usually greater than that for psoriasis elsewhere. Disease on the palms improves by about 10 treatments and clears by 30 treatments, while disease on the soles improves by 15 treatments and may require up to 40 treatments for clearance. The doses of UVA radiation required to achieve clearance on the palms are about 25% higher and on the soles about 50% higher than comparable whole-body doses.

Topical PUVA Therapy

Application of a psoralen solution and use of a psoralen bath have been reported as useful alternatives to systemic therapy and have yielded comparable rates of clearance. Use of the solution is associated with prolonged photosensitivity and recurrent phototoxicity, which are significant problems. However, the soaking approach appears to avoid these problems. The hands or feet are soaked for 30 min in 2 L of water containing 1 mL of 1% methoxsalen solution, dried, and immediately exposed to 1 J/cm^2 of UVA radiation with increments of 0.5 J/cm^2 each treatment as tolerated.

Maintenance Therapy

When a patient is cleared of disease on the palms and soles, maintenance therapy can be given on a similar schedule as for whole-body treatment. However, if a patient is only partially cleared, long-term maintenance is usually required to control symptoms, and this particularly applies to disease on the soles since the clearance rate at this site is lower.

PSORIASIS OF THE NAILS

Nature of the Disease

Psoriasis of the nails usually occurs in association with psoriasis of the skin and the patients' focus is on their skin disease. However, sometimes patients are very concerned about the pitting, dystrophy, or onycholysis on their fingernails and request treatment. In addition, occasionally a patient presents with extensive fingernail psoriasis and minimal or no disease elsewhere.

Management

Oral PUVA Therapy

Fingernail psoriasis does respond in some patients during whole-body treatment. In one study we observed that patients with nail involvement did not clear their nails by the end of a clearance course for their skin disease but after 4 months of maintenance therapy, 60% had resolution of their nail disease and there were no differences in the response rates between pitting, dystrophy, and onycholysis. Patients in this study were not given local treatment to the hands. This response rate can be improved to about 75% if patients are given extra treatments to the hands in addition to whole-body treatment for cutaneous psoriasis. In patients with nail disease alone who are greatly disturbed by their condition and very motivated, treatment to just the dorsa of the hands may be considered. However, it is important for the patient to understand that clearance will take 4–6 months, the rate of success is about 75%, and recurrence is likely in the absence of maintenance treatment. Improvement in disease of the toenails does not occur during regular treatment of the feet, so attempts to treat this problem are probably futile.

Topical PUVA Therapy

Application of 1% methoxsalen solution to the proximal nail fold up to the terminal phalanx followed by exposure to UVA radiation was successful in clearing some patients with pitting and onycholysis in a small study.

BIBLIOGRAPHY

Abel EA, Goldberg LH, Farber EM. Treatment of palmoplantar psoriasis with topical methoxsalen plus long-wave ultraviolet light. Arch Dermatol 1980; 116:1257–1261.

Agren-Jonsson S, Tegner E. PUVA therapy for palmoplantar pustulosis. Acta Dermatol 1985; 65:531–535.

Coleman WR, Lowe NJ, David M, Halder RM. Palmoplantar psoriasis: experience with 8-methoxypsoralen soaks plus ultraviolet A with the use of a high-output metal halide device. J Am Acad Dermatol 1989; 20:1078–1082.

Hawk JLM, Grice PL. The efficacy of localized PUVA therapy for chronic hand and foot dermatoses. Clin and Exp Dermatol 1994; 19: 479–482.

Hönigsmann H, Gschnait F, Konrad K, Wolff K. Photochemotherapy for pustular psoriasis. Br J Dermatol 1977; 97:119–126.

Jansen CT, Malmiharju T. Inefficacy of topical methoxsalen plus UVA for palmoplantar pustulosis. Acta Dermatol 1981; 61:354–356.

Lassus A, Lauharanta J, Eskelinen A. The effect of etretinate compared with different regimens of PUVA in the treatment of persistent palmo-plantar pustulosis. Br J Dermatol 1985; 112:455–459.

Lawrence CM, Marks J, Parker S, Shuster S. A comparison of PUVA-etre-tinate and PUVA-placebo for palmoplantar pustular psoriasis. Br J Dermatol 1984; 110:221–226.

Mobacken H, Rosen K, Swanbeck G. Oral psoralen photochemotherapy (PUVA) of hyperkeratotic dermatitis of the palms. Br J Dermatol 1983; 109:205–208.

Morison WL, Parrish JA, Fitzpatrick TB. Oral methoxsalen photoche-motherapy of recalcitrant dermatoses of the palms and soles. Br J Dermatol 1978; 99:297–302.

Murray D, Corbett WF, Warin AP. A controlled trial of photochemother-apy for persistent palmoplantar pustulosis. Br J Dermatol 1980; 102:659.

Paul R, Jansen CT. Suppression of palmoplantar pustulosis symptoms with oral 8-methoxypsoralen and high-intensity UVA irradiation. Derma-tologica. 1983; 167:283–285.

Vukas A. Photochemotherapy in treatment of psoriatic variants. Dermato-logica 1977; 155:355–361.

Wilkinson JD, Ralfs ID, Harper JI, Black MM. Topical methoxsalen photo-chemotherapy in the treatment of palmoplantar pustulosis and psoriasis. Acta Dermatol 1979; 59:193–198.

15

Eczema

INTRODUCTION

UV therapy is widely used in the treatment of eczema and is generally employed as a second-line treatment after failure of topical therapy. Atopic eczema has been the disease evaluated in most studies of UV therapy since it is common and represents a fairly uniform disease. This focus on atopic eczema, however, should not obscure the fact that most eczemas can be successfully treated with UV therapy.

There is an important distinction between the goal of successful conservative topical therapy and the goal of successful UV therapy. Topical therapy is aimed at reducing inflammation and pruritus but it seldom totally suppresses eczema, or if it does, it seldom remains in remission for long. UV therapy should be aimed at achieving and maintaining a remission free of disease because only then is it possible to have a long remission off all treatment.

INDICATIONS FOR THERAPY

The main indications for UV therapy are listed in Table 1. The first two indications are to some extent intertwined since a patient may have a good response to topical therapy, but for the patient this response may be inadequate since his or her desire is to be cleared of eczema. Extensive disease and even erythroderma can respond to UV therapy so that topical therapy becomes adjunctive therapy and UV therapy is a first-line treatment. Pityriasis alba is a special situation where again UV therapy should be the

Table 1 Indications for UV Therapy

Failure of topical therapy
Desire of patient to be free of eczema
Extensive disease
Steroid-sparing agent
Pityriasis alba

---

first-line treatment since it will suppress the eczema and also restore normal pigmentation. Use of UV therapy for its steroid-sparing effect can be important at all ages, particularly in patients who have the required multiple courses of oral steroids. However, it is particularly important in the child or adolescent with growth retardation from heavy exposure to corticosteroids and a switch to UV therapy will often be associated with a spurt in growth.

ATOPIC ECZEMA

Various types of UV therapy have been used to treat atopic eczema and although there have been only a few comparative studies the order of treatments in terms of efficacy appears to be oral or topical PUVA therapy, narrow-band UVB phototherapy, broad-band UVA/UVB, and broad-band UVB phototherapy.

Oral PUVA Therapy

Clearance Treatment

This is the most effective form of UV therapy and can be used in patients with moderate involvement through to erythrodermic disease. A T.I.W. or 11011 schedule gives the best results, and 30–50 treatments are usually required to achieve satisfactory control of disease. Control of disease means the body surface is free of any evidence of the disease. The first sign of improvement is a decrease in pruritus, and this may occur after only a few treatments. However, improvement of the rash may not begin to occur until after 20 or more treatments.

Maintenance Treatment

Maintenance therapy is not only essential but also must be more aggressive and rigid than in the case of psoriasis. In patients with atopic eczema, a miss of one or two treatments in the early part of the maintenance phase, may result in a rapid return of whole-body eczema, as compared to a slow return of the disease with psoriasis. Pruritus is the first symptom of a flare-up of the disease and precedes the appearance of eczema by several days; the appearance of this symptom is an indication to increase the frequency of treatment. Atopic eczema patients initially require weekly treatments for maintenance therapy, but this requirement for such intensive therapy does decrease with time.

Results of Treatment

The results achieved when using PUVA as a monotherapy very much depend on the patients being treated. Clearance rates of more than 90% are possible in patients with moderate disease, particularly if it is of short duration. These patients can then be maintained clear for a few months and then treatment can be stopped and they usually have a long remission. The clearance rate for patients with severe disease, particularly if it is of long duration, is < 50%. Furthermore, more than half of these patients fail maintenance treatment and have significant exacerbations of their disease. Combination therapy is often required to clear and maintain patients with severe atopic eczema.

Narrow-Band UVB Phototherapy

Narrow-band UVB phototherapy is mainly indicated for patients with mild or moderate disease. However, it can be used in younger patients with more severe disease as an alternative to oral PUVA therapy.

Clearance Treatment

A T.I.W. schedule is essential since B.I.W. treatment is seldom successful. Patients are started at 70% of their MED and the dose is increased 10%, 15%, or 20% each treatment depending on the response and severity of the disease. As with PUVA therapy, pruritus responds before improvement in the rash, which may not start to clear until after 15–20 treatments. Clearance often requires 30–50 treatments.

Maintenance Treatment

A period of maintenance therapy is always required starting with B.I.W. treatment and then reducing to QW treatment after a couple of months.

Results of Treatment

When treating mild to moderate disease a clearance rate of 75% or higher is possible and most of these patients can stop maintenance therapy after a few months and have a long remission. The response rate in severe disease is much lower but a trial of this treatment is worthwhile in younger patients.

Broad-Band UVB/UVA Phototherapy

Several studies indicate that combined exposure to both broad-band UVA and broad-band UVB radiation is effective in mild to moderate atopic eczema and is superior to broad-band UVB radiation alone.

Clearance Treatment

Three to five treatments are required each week starting with 70% of the MED_{UVB} and increasing this dose by 20% each treatment to maintain an erythemogenic schedule. The starting dose of UVA radiation is 10 J/cm^2 and this can be increased by 1 J/cm^2 each treatment up to 20 J/cm^2. As an alternative, if UVA radiation is not available, the same doses of UVB radiation can be given as a monotherapy.

Maintenance Treatment

Maintenance treatment is required and can be given as B.I.W. treatment for a few months and then as QW treatment.

Results of Treatment

Most patients with mild to moderate eczema will be considerably improved by this treatment but only a minority will be cleared of disease.

HAND ECZEMA

Eczema confined to the hands is often resistant to topical therapy and since it is a cause of significant physical and social disability, UV therapy is often a treatment of choice.

Hand eczema in adults does not respond to either broad-band or narrow-band UVB phototherapy and should be treated with topical or oral PUVA therapy. The problem is simply optical. UVB photons do not penetrate the thickened epidermis of the palms in sufficient amounts to clear eczema at this site. The exception to this is young children with thin eczema and minimal scaliness who may respond to narrow-band UVB phototherapy.

Oral PUVA Therapy

A regular schedule as for psoriasis is used with exposure to UVA radiation in a hand and foot unit or if this is not available, the hands can be exposed to one bank of a stand-up unit with the remainder of the body covered. A T.I.W. schedule is best and the aim is total clearance.

Table 2 Response of Hand Eczema to PUVA Therapy

Very responsive
Atopic
Dyshidrotic
Fingertip
Responsive
Chronic irritant
Hyperkeratotic
Unresponsive
Allergic contact

Topical PUVA Therapy

Application of a psoralen solution or soaking the hands in a weak solution of psoralen is an alternative approach and comparable rates of clearance are achieved.

Results of Treatment

The clearance rates and the number of treatments required to achieve clearance depend on the type of eczema being treated (Table 2). Atopic, dyshidrotic, and fingertip eczema begin to improve by treatment 10 and most patients are clear after 25–30 treatments. Chronic irritant dermatitis as seen in hairdressers, and other people involved in a lot of wet work or in contact with other irritants are slow to clear and may require 50 or more treatments to clear. Hyperkeratotic eczema is also slow to clear and keratolytics should be used. If improvement is not apparent in any patient with hand eczema by treatment 20, allergic contact eczema should be considered and appropriate patch testing be done. Allergic contact dermatitis does not respond to PUVA therapy.

Maintenance Treatment

A period of maintenance treatment is always required starting with weekly treatments and gradually reducing to monthly treatments. The duration of maintenance treatment is roughly proportional to the length of the clearance phase with a minimum of about 6 months.

OTHER ECZEMAS

Various other types of eczema respond to UV therapy and the choice of treatment and the likely response largely depend on the type of eczema (Table 3).

Table 3 Response of Other Eczemas to UV Therapy

Very responsive
Pityriasis alba
Asteatotic eczema
Responsive
Nummular eczema
Seborrhoeic eczema
Slow response
Prurigo nodularis

Pityriasis Alba

Widespread pityriasis alba is most common in children and adolescents but does occur in adults. It occurs in all races but is particularly a problem in African–Americans. PUVA therapy is the treatment of choice and it clears in as few as 10 treatments. Narrow-band UVB phototherapy is also effective but about twice as many treatments are required, probably because it is less effective in suppressing inflammation and in stimulating melanogenesis. Maintenance treatment can be given for a couple of months.

Asteatotic or Winter Eczema

This condition has many names but is usually seen in older patients in cold climates particularly in people who love soap and long, hot showers or baths. Correcting these habits and liberal use of moisturizers are certainly part of the treatment but UV therapy can produce rapid clearance in 10–20 treatments. Both PUVA therapy and UVB phototherapy are effective and maintenance requirements are minimal.

Nummular Eczema

The choice of treatment in this condition will depend on the degree of inflammation and infiltration or thickness of the lesions. Thinner lesions will respond to UVB phototherapy while thicker, more inflamed lesions suggest use of PUVA therapy. Clearance is usually easy to achieve but recurrences are common and prolonged maintenance is often required.

Seborrhoeic Dermatitis

The generalized form of this condition responds to PUVA therapy in a manner similar to atopic eczema with the response being determined by the amount of inflammation present. Prolonged maintenance for as long as a year is often required.

Table 4 Combination Therapies

PUVA/broad-band UVB therapy
Long-term corticosteroids
Steroid-sparing agents
Methotrexate
Azathioprine
Mycophenolate mofetil

Prurigo Nodularis

Widespread prurigo nodularis responds to PUVA therapy but the response is slow. Improvement begins after about 20 treatments and clearance requires 50–75 treatments. However, if total clearance is achieved and the patient receives a few months of maintenance, the recurrence rate is low.

ADJUNCTIVE TREATMENT

Patients must continue their current regimen of topical or systemic corticosteroids until their eczema begins to respond to PUVA or UV phototherapy, at which time these treatments can be gradually reduced. Stopping these treatments prior to therapy will only produce a rebound exacerbation and possible failure of treatment. However, the exception to this is use of topical immunomodulators such as tacrolimus and pimecrolimus. These agents should be stopped before commencing UV therapy because their potential role in increasing the risk of skin cancer is still being defined.

COMBINATION THERAPY

Some patients cannot be cleared of their eczema or be maintained in a clear state using UV treatment as a monotherapy and the use of combination therapy has to be considered (Table 4).

PUVA/Broadband UVB Therapy

This is a simple combination treatment, which should be considered as the initial clearance treatment in any patient with a high skin type (IV–VI) and any patient with severe eczema. In addition, it is useful in patients who are slow to respond to PUVA therapy. In such patients, broad-band UVB treatment can be added in a starting dose of 0.030 J/cm^2 (skin type I) up to 0.100 J/cm^2 (skin type VI) with increments of 20% in each treatment. Use of this combination in maintenance failures who are skin types I–III is intensive due to loss of tolerance to the UVB component and treatment cannot be reduced to less than QW or Q2W frequency.

Table 5 Problems of Therapy

Exacerbations during clearance phase
Psychological factors
Folliculitis
Dry skin
Depigmentation
Herpes simplex

Long-Term Corticosteroids

This is a tempting combination with UV therapy, particularly in patients who are already on these agents. However, the risk of adverse effects is high and careful monitoring is required.

Steroid-Sparing Agents

Several systemic agents have been reported as being beneficial in eczema and can be considered for use in combination with UV therapy. These include methotrexate, azathioprine, and mycophenolate mofetil. Cyclosporin should not be used because of the increased risk of skin cancer.

PROBLEMS OF THERAPY

There are several problems unique to the treatment of eczema (Table 5).

Exacerbations during the Clearance Phase

This is the single most important problem in treating eczema with UV therapy. It is a problem for the physician if it is not understood and for the patients if they have not been warned ahead of time before treatment is started. When treating most other diseases with UV therapy, improvement begins early after a few treatments, and steady improvement is seen thereafter. This pattern of response does not occur in eczema. Improvement is often delayed and may not begin until treatment 20, particularly in patients with severe disease, but is then quite rapid. If the patients are going to have an exacerbation of their eczema before the effect of treatment begins they will still have that exacerbation despite being on treatment. This we observed in bilateral comparison studies where one side was not treated and exacerbations occurred on both sides. The patient interprets the exacerbation as being due to treatment and the physician may come to the same conclusion if he is not aware of this phenomenon.

There are two approaches to this problem. The physician can try to convince the patient to continue treatment and that the treatment is not the cause of the problem. Alternatively, a brief course of oral corticosteroids can be given while continuing treatment. Prednisone in a dose of 60 mg daily for 10 days and then reducing the dose to zero over the next 12 days is suitable for most patients. The mental health of the patient and the physician dictates the choice between the two approaches.

Psychological Factors

Psychological factors appear to be very important in determining the response to treatment for both the short- and the long-term outlook. Patients who are poorly adjusted to their disease tend to show a poor response to UV therapy and, if cleared of disease, frequently relapse. Therefore, it is important to assess the motivation and psychological state of the patient before beginning the treatment. Patients with atopic eczema differ from psoriatic patients in that they are more questioning, anxious, and introverted. As a result, they require much more support and, hence, more physician time.

Folliculitis

Folliculitis or other evidence of secondary infection is common in patients with atopic eczema. Oral antibiotics are necessary if folliculitis is a problem since this does not respond to UV therapy and its persistence can lead to an exacerbation of eczema. A few patients require rotating antibiotics to control this problem.

Dry Skin

Moisturizers must be used by all patients since dry skin is often associated with eczema and UV therapy accentuates this problem.

Depigmentation

Depigmentation is a common sequela after clearance of areas of chronic lichenification, and this complicates dosimetry because the exposure dose required to maintain control of normally pigmented skin exceeds the erythema threshold of the white skin. Application of a broad-spectrum sunscreen to the depigmented area prior to treatment is a rather inexact solution to the problem. Repigmentation may occur but this can take a year or more of therapy.

Herpes Simplex

Disseminated or ophthalmic herpes simplex is a theoretical risk but only one case of each condition has been observed, and in both instances treatment was continued after appropriate therapy for the simplex infection.

BIBLIOGRAPHY

Atopic Eczema

PUVA Therapy

Morison WL, Parrish JA, Fitzpatrick TB. Oral psoralen photochemotherapy of atopic eczema. Br J Dermatol 1978; 98:25–30.

Morris AD, Saihan EM. Maintenance psoralen plus ultraviolet A therapy: does it have a role in the treatment of severe atopic eczema? Br J Dermatol 2002; 146:705–718.

Ogawa H, Yoshiike T. Atopic dermatitis: studies of skin permeability and effectiveness of topical PUVA treatment. Pediatr Dermatol 1992; 9: 383–385.

Sannwald C, Ortonne JP, Thivolet J. La photochimiothérapie orale de l'eczéma atopique. Dermatologica 1979; 159:71–77.

Sheehan MP, Atherton DJ, Norris P, Hawk J. Oral psoralen photochemotherapy in severe childhood atopic eczema: an update. Br J Dermatol 1993; 129:431–436.

Soppi E, Viander M, Soppi AM, Jansén CT. Cell-mediated immunity in untreated and PUVA treated atopic dermatitis. J Invest Dermatol 1982; 79:213–217.

Zaynoun S, Javer LAA, Kurban AK. Oral methoxsalen photochemotherapy of extensive pityriasis alba. J Am Acad Dermatol 1986; 15: 61–65.

Narrowband UVB Phototherapy

Collins P, Ferguson J. Narrowband (TL-01) UVB air-conditioned phototherapy for atopic eczema in children. Br J Dermatol 1995; 133:653–667.

Der-Petrossian M, Seeber A, Hönigsmann H, Tanew A. Half-side comparison study on the efficacy of 8-methoxypsoralen bath-PUVA versus narrow-band ultraviolet B phototherapy in patients with severe chronic atopic dermatitis. Br J Dermatol 2000; 142:39–43.

George SA, Bilsland DJ, Johnson BE, Ferguson J. Narrow-band (TL-01) UVB air-conditioned phototherapy for chronic severe adult atopic dermatitis. Br J Dermatol 1993; 128:49–56.

Grundmann-Kollmann M, Behrens S, Podda M, Peter RU, Kaufmann R, Kerscher M. Phototherapy for atopic eczema with narrow-band UVB. J Am Acad Dermatol 1999; 40:995–997.

Hudson-Peacock MJ, Diffey BL, Farr PM. Narrow-band UVB phototherapy for severe atopic dermatitis. Br J Dermatol 1996; 135:332.

Legat FJ, Hofer A, Brabek E, Quehenberger F, Kerl H, Wolf P. Narrowband UV-B vs medium-dose UV-A1 phototherapy in chronic atopic dermatitis. Arch Dermatol 2003; 139:223–224.

Broad-Band UVB and UVA/UVB Therapy

Falk ES. UV-light therapies in atopic dermatitis. Photodermatology 1985; 2:241–246.

Hannuksela M, Karvonen J, Husa M, Jokela R, Katajamäki L, Leppisaari M. Ultraviolet light therapy in atopic dermatitis. Acta Dermatol Venereol 1985; 114:137–139.

Jekler J, Larkö O. UVB phototherapy of atopic dermatitis. Br J Dermatol 1988; 119:697–705.

Jekler J, Larkö O. The effect of ultraviolet radiation with peaks at 300 nm and 350 nm in the treatment of atopic dermatitis. Photodermatol Photoimmunol Photomed 1990; 7:169–172.

Jekler J, Larkö O. Combined UVA–UVB versus UVB phototherapy for atopic dermatitis: a paired-comparison study. J Am Acad Dermatol 1990; 22:49–53.

Jekler J, Larkö O. Phototherapy for atopic dermatitis with ultraviolet A (UVA), low-dose UVB, and combined UVA and UVB: two paired-comparison studies. Photodermatol Photoimmunol Photomed 1991; 8:151–156.

Midelfart K, Stenvold SE, Volden G. Combined UVB and UVA phototherapy of atopic eczema. Dermatologica 1985; 171:95–98.

Wulf HC, Bech-Thomsen N. A UVB phototherapy protocol with very low dose increments as a treatment of atopic dermatitis. Photodermatol Photoimmunol Photomed 1998; 14:1–6.

Hand Eczema

LeVine MJ, Parrish JA, Fitzpatrick TB. Oral methoxsalen photochemotherapy (PUVA) of dyshidrotic eczema. Acta Dermatol Venereol 1981; 61: 570–571.

Mobacken H, Rosen K, Swanbeck G. Oral psoralen photochemotherapy (PUVA) of hyperkeratotic dermatitis of the palms. Br J Dermatol 1983; 109:205–208.

Sheehan-Dare RA, Goodfield MJ, Rowell NR. Topical psoralen photochemotherapy (PUVA) and superficial radiotherapy in the treatment of chronic hand eczema. Br J Dermatol 1989; 121:65–69.

Sjövall P, Christensen OB. Local and systemic effect of UVB irradiation in patients with chronic hand eczema. Acta Dermatol Venereol 1987; 67:538–541.

Tegner E, Thelin I. PUVA treatment of chronic eczematous dermatitis of the palms and soles. Acta Dermatol Venereol 1985; 65:451–453.

Other Eczemas

Dahl KB, Reymann F. Photochemotherapy in erythrodermic seborrhoic dermatitis. Arch Dermatol 1977; 113:1295–1296.

Hann SK, Cho MY, Park YK. UV treatment of generalized prurigo nodularis. Int J Dermatol 1990; 29:436–437.

Pirkhammer D, Seeber A, Hönigsmann H, Tanew A. Narrow-band ultraviolet B (TL-01) phototherapy is an effective and safe treatment option for patients with severe seborrhoeic dermatitis. Br J Dermatol 2000; 143:964–968.

Väätäinen N, Hannuksela M, Karvonen J. Local photochemotherapy in nodular prurigo. Acta Dermatol Venereol 1979; 59:544–547.

16

Mycosis Fungoides

INTRODUCTION

Mycosis fungoides is the most common of the cutaneous T-cell lymphomas, a group of disorders that arise from malignant $CD4^+$ helper T cells and localize within skin and associated lymph nodes. Mycosis fungoides is often preceded by a benign phase, which may last years and is usually diagnosed as a nonspecific eczema. Thus, diagnosis is often delayed and even when the diagnosis is considered, histologic confirmation may not be possible. Due to its varying presentations and biologic behavior there is still much uncertainty as to what is the best management for mycosis fungoides but there does appear to be general consensus that UV therapy has a significant role in the management of the early stages of disease.

INDICATIONS FOR UV THERAPY

Primary Treatment

UV therapy is suitable as a primary treatment in the patch and plaque stage of the disease in the absence of lymph node or visceral lymphoma. This corresponds to stages 1A, 1B, and IIA of one frequently used classification of mycosis fungoides (Table 1). In addition, UV therapy may be used in the premalignant phase of the disease when the diagnosis is suspected but cannot be confirmed. This phase is often labeled as parapsoriasis en plaque.

Table 1 Staging of Early Mycosis Fungoides

Stage	Skin involvement	Lymph node
IA	<10% BSA[a]	
IB	>10% BSA	
IIA	Variable area	Palpable, pathology negative
IIB	One or more tumors	Palpable, pathology negative

[a]BSA, body surface area.

Palliative Treatment

UV therapy may be used as a palliative treatment in the IIB tumor stage provided some additional treatment such as radiotherapy is given for the tumors; these patients tend to have progressive disease and control of the skin disease is seldom achieved. UV therapy can also be useful in advanced disease (stages III and IV) with visceral involvement since clearance of skin disease improves quality of life.

DIAGNOSIS, EVALUATION, AND STAGING OF DISEASE

Diagnosis

A definite diagnosis must be made. Often in early stages of the disease the clinical picture may be consistent with mycosis fungoides but the histopathology is not diagnostic. In these patients multiple biopsy samples of skin should be obtained. Immunophenotyping of the cutaneous infiltrate to identify T-cell subsets and examination of T-cell receptor gene rearrangement by PCR studies are often helpful in establishing the diagnosis.

Evaluation and Staging

Accurate staging of disease is important because this will dictate choice of treatment and ultimate prognosis. These steps are outlined in Table 2.

PUVA THERAPY

Oral PUVA therapy has been used in several ways for treatment of early stages of mycosis fungoides. The commonest approach is to use a clearance course, with or without histologic confirmation of clearance, followed by limited maintenance treatment over a few months. This approach gives long-term remissions of years in 30–50% of patients. Those patients who relapse will usually respond to a further course of treatment. This is certainly a good approach in patients with parapsoriasis or the premalignant phase of the disease.

Table 2 Evaluation and Staging of Disease

History and physical examination
  Extent and type of skin disease
  Palpation of peripheral lymph nodes
Laboratory investigations
  Complete blood count
  Liver function tests
  Sezary cell count
If lymph nodes are palpable
  Node biopsy
  Chest x-ray
  CT abdomen and pelvis
If Sezary count is positive
  Bone marrow aspiration

An alternative approach which I use is based on two premises. First, mycosis fungoides is a potentially lethal neoplasm and should not be treated as a benign dermatosis. Second, there is no definite evidence that PUVA therapy is ever curative in mycosis fungoides, but there is evidence that it can control disease. The regimen is outlined in Table 3.

Clearance Schedule

Several studies have shown that atypical cells can still be present in the dermis when the skin is completely clear on clinical examination, so the end point for clearance should be total clinical and histological clearance of disease. If atypical cells are still present on the first biopsies, another 10 treatments are given and the biopsies repeated. About 95% of patients with early disease can be cleared in 20–40 treatments with the slower clearance likely to occur in those with extensive disease and thicker plaques. If total clearance is not achieved, consideration should be given to trying combination treatment.

Table 3 PUVA Therapy for Mycosis Fungoides

Clearance treatment (TIW or 11011) until clinically clear of disease
Ten more treatments on clearance schedule at held dose of UVA: two biopsies next
  to previous positive biopsies
Histologically clear: switch to maintenance
  QW for 6 months
  Q2W for 6 months
  QM forever

Maintenance Phase

The necessity and rationale for long-term treatment must be explained to the patient at the beginning of therapy. Any evidence of recurrent disease requires a return to clearance treatment and adjustment of the frequency of exposures and doses as required.

NARROWBAND UVB PHOTOTHERAPY

There have been several studies of the use of narrowband UVB phototherapy in patients with stages IA and IB mycosis fungoides. The main concerns with using this modality in mycosis fungoides are twofold. Due to lack of penetration by UVB radiation, atypical cells in the deeper portion of the dermis are unlikely to be removed. Second, maintenance treatment is not really practical due to the requirement of a high frequency of treatment. However, for patients with very slowly progressive disease, very early disease or, if there is a contraindication to using PUVA therapy, narrowband phototherapy may be a useful option.

Clearance Schedule

Three or more treatments per week are required and clearance rates of 50–80% of patients have been reported in 20–40 treatments. However, the definition often used for a complete response is more than 95% clear or minimal residual disease. In addition histologic clearance of atypical cells is often not observed. The duration of a remission varies but probably averages about 6 months with a range of 2–12 months.

Intermittent Therapy

An option when using narrowband phototherapy is to give repeated courses of clearance therapy and this option needs to be evaluated in a prospective study. Whether or not it is successful in a given patient depends on duration of the clearance course, duration of the remission, and how well the disease continues to respond to treatment.

BROADBAND UVB PHOTOTHERAPY

There are two reports that broadband UVB phototherapy, mainly used as home phototherapy, can clear patch stage mycosis fungoides in about 70% of cases although this required many months of treatment. Some patients did have long remissions after stopping treatment. Plaque stage disease did not respond.

COMBINATION THERAPY

Combination therapy should be considered in the following patients:

- High skin type
- Extensive disease or thick plaques
- Disease in sanctuary areas such as scalp and intertriginous areas
- Failure to clear with UV therapy alone.

PUVA/Broadband UVB Phototherapy

This is a useful combination treatment as an initial therapy in patients with skin types IV–VI. It is also useful in hypopigmented mycosis fungoides, an uncommon form of the disease which occurs in more pigmented patients and can be difficult to clear.

PUVA/Retinoids

A course of acitretin (1 mg/kg body weight daily) started 2 weeks before commencing PUVA therapy can lower the number of treatments required and cumulative exposure dose of UVA radiation but the percentage of patients cleared is not increased. Maintenance options vary but continuation of PUVA therapy alone is probably the simplest approach.

PUVA/Interferon Alpha-2a

There is good evidence from several studies that a combination of PUVA plus interferon alpha-2a (Roferon®) given intramuscularly or subcutaneously is a combination treatment superior to either treatment alone. It can be used as a primary treatment at any stage of the disease but is probably not justified in stage IA since these patients respond well to PUVA therapy alone and the marked side effects of interferon cause considerable morbidity. The response rate is the best in early-stage disease (IB, IIA) and more advanced stages have a lower rate of complete responses. The combination therapy is useful in patients who have failed to clear with PUVA therapy alone. The dose of interferon used has varied from 6 million units daily to 30 million units three times a week with the higher doses being associated with more side effects. At high interferon doses, photosensitivity in the form of unexpected erythema can be a problem in nearly a third of patients. Therefore, when using a high dose of interferon (>50 million units per week) a conservative approach should be taken with both the initial dose of UVA radiation and escalation of this dose. Lower doses of interferon do not appear to be associated with photosensitivity.

PUVA/Topical Nitrogen Mustard

Combining PUVA therapy with nitrogen mustard treatment has the advantage of treating sanctuary sites in relatively unexposed areas. However, combining two carcinogenic treatments probably increases the risk of skin cancer. There is no evidence that PUVA therapy decreases the frequency of contact allergy to nitrogen mustard.

PUVA/Electron Beam Therapy

Recurrent disease following total body electron beam treatment has been successfully treated with PUVA therapy but this combination should be avoided for two reasons. First, it is combining two carcinogenic treatments and a high frequency of various skin cancers has been observed in these patients. Second, rapid development of photoaging of the skin can occur with this sequence of treatments, particularly in patients with a low skin type.

PUVA/Bexarotene

This combination has been used in patients who failed monotherapy with early, intermediate, and advanced (Sezary syndrome) stages of disease with control of disease in most patients. There were no particular problems with the combination and it deserves further study.

PHOTOSENSITIVITY

Photosensitivity is common in patients with mycosis fungoides and it may appear in various forms during the course of UV therapy.

Abnormal Phototesting

Increased sensitivity to UVB, UVA, and sometimes visible light may be detected in as many as 20% of patients when phototested on normal skin. This does not usually interfere with treatment except that lower doses of UVA or UVB are tolerated during PUVA or narrowband UVB therapy. In a few patients the photosensitivity is marked and has to be suppressed by a short course of prednisone so that UV therapy can continue. The protocol given for treatment of chronic photosensitivity is suitable in these patients.

Photosensitivity Confined to Lesions

A few patients develop erythema and sometimes blisters confined to lesional skin after the first few UV treatments. Cessation of treatment until the reaction settles and then use of reduced doses of radiation usually circumvents this problem. This is usually a good prognostic sign since these patients tend to clear more rapidly than unaffected patients.

Exacerbation of Disease

A few patients, early in the course of UV treatment, usually after three or four exposures, develop an extensive exacerbation of their disease with dozens of new lesions on previously, at least clinically, uninvolved skin. There is usually no background erythema and phototesting of normal skin will give normal results. Treatment should not be stopped but the usual increases in dose should be continued, and again the prognosis for a rapid clearance is usually excellent.

BIBLIOGRAPHY

Staging

Demierre MF, Foss FM, Koh HK. Proceedings of the international consensus conference on cutaneous T-cell lymphoma (CTCL) treatment recommendations. J Am Acad Dermatol 1997; 36:460–466.

PUVA Therapy

Abel EA, Deneau DG, Farber EM, Price NM, Hoppe RT. PUVA treatment of erythrodermic and plaque type mycosis fungoides. J Am Acad Dermatol 1981; 4:423–429.

Akarphanth R, Douglass MC, Lim HW. Hypopigmented mycosis fungoides: treatment and a 6-1/2 year follow-up of 9 patients. J Am Acad Dermatol 2000; 42:33–39.

Briffa DV, Warin AP, Harrington CI, Bleehan SS. Photochemotherapy in mycosis fungoides. Lancet 1980; 2:49–53.

Child FJ, Mitchell TJ, Whittaker SJ, Scarisbrick JJ, Seed PT, Russell-Jones R. A randomized cross-over study to compare PUVA and extracorporeal photopheresis in the treatment of plaque stage (T2) mycosis fungoides. Clin Exp Dermatol 2004; 29:231–236.

ischer T, Skogh M. Treatment of parapsoriasis en plaques, mycosis fungoides, and Sezary's syndrome with trioxsalen baths followed by ultraviolet light. Acta Dermatol Venereol (Stockh) 1979; 59:171–173.

Gilchrest BA, Parrish JA, Tanenbaum L, Haynes HA, Fitzpatrick TB. Oral methoxsalen photochemotherapy of mycosis fungoides. Cancer 1976; 38:683–689.

Herrmann JJ, Roenigk HH, Hurria A, Kuzel TM, Samuelson E, Rademaker AW, Rosen ST. Treatment of mycosis fungoides with photochemotherapy (PUVA): long-term follow-up. J Am Acad Dermatol 1995; 33:234–342.

Hönigsmann H, Tanew A, Wolff K. Treatment of mycosis fungoides with PUVA. Photodermatology 1987; 4:55–58.

Hönigsman H, Brenner W, Rauschmeier W, Konrad K, Wolff K. Photochemotherapy for cutaneous T cell lymphoma. J Am Acad Dermatol 1984; 10:238–245.

Kaye FJ, Bunn PA, Steinberg SM, Stocker JL, Ihde DC, Fischmann AB, Glatstein EJ, Schechter GP, Phelps RM, Foss FM, Parlette HL, Anderson MJ, Sausville EA. A randomized trial comparing combination electron-beam radiation and chemotherapy with topical therapy in the initial treatment of mycosis fungoides. N Engl J Med 1989; 321:1784–1790.

Mackie RM, Foulds IS, McMillan EM, Nelson HM. Histological changes observed in the skin of patients with mycosis fungoides receiving photochemotherapy. Clin Exp Dermatol 1980; 5:405–413.

Molin L, Thomsen K, Volden G, Groth O. Photochemotherapy (PUVA) in the pretumour stage of mycosis fungoides: a report from the Scandinavian mycosis fungoides study group. Acta Dermatol Venereol (Stockh) 1980; 61:47–51.

Pabsch H, Rütten A, von Stemm A, Meigel W, Sander CA, Schaller J. Treatment of childhood mycosis fungoides with topical PUVA. J Am Acad Dermatol 2002; 47:557–561.

Roenigk HH. Photochemotherapy for mycosis fungoides. Arch Dermatol 1977; 113:1047–1051.

Roupe G, Sandström MH, Kjellström C. PUVA in early mycosis fungoides may give long-term remission and delay extracutaneous spread. Acta Dermatol Venereol (Stockh) 1996; 76:475–478.

Swanbeck G, Roupe G, Sandström MH. Indications of a considerable decrease in the death rate in mycosis fungoides by PUVA treatment. Acta Dermatol Venereol (Stockh) 1994; 74: 465–466.

Whitmore SE, Simmons-O'Brien E, Rotter FS. Hypopigmented mycosis fungoides. Arch Dermatol 1994; 130:476–480.

Narrowband UVB Phototherapy

Clark C, Dawe RS, Evans AT, Lowe G, Ferguson J. Narrowband TL-01 phototherapy for patch-stage mycosis fungoides. Arch Dermatol 2000; 136: 748–752.

Gathers RC, Scherschun L, Malick F, Fivenson DP, Lim HW. Narrowband UVB phototherapy for early-stage mycosis fungoides. J Am Acad Dermatol 2002; 47:191–197.

Hofer A, Cerroni L, Kerl H, Wolf P. Narrowband (311-nm) UV-B therapy for small plaque parapsoriasis and early-stage mycosis fungoides. Arch Dermatol 1999; 135:1377–1380.

Pascale V, Diederen MM, van Weelden H, Sanders CJG, Toonstra J, van Vloten WA. Narrowband UVB and psoralen-UVA in the treatment of early-stage mycosis fungoides: a retrospective study. J Am Acad Dermatol 2003; 48:215–219.

Broadband UVB Phototherapy

Ramsay DL, Lish KM, Yalowitz CB, Soter NA. Ultraviolet-B phototherapy for early-stage cutaneous T-cell lymphoma. Arch Dermatol 1992; 128:931–933.
Resnik KS, Vonderheid EC. Home UV phototherapy of early mycosis fungoides: long-term follow-up observations in thirty-one patients. J Am Acad Dermatol 1993; 29:73–77.

Combination Therapy—Retinoids

Thomsen K, Hammar H, Molin L, Volden G. Retinoids plus PUVA (RePUVA) in mycosis fungoides, plaque stage. Acta Dermatol Venereol (Stockh) 1989; 69:536–538.

Combination Therapy—Interferon

Chang LW, Liranzo M, Bergfeld WF. Cutaneous side effects associated with interferon-alpha therapy: a review. Cutis 1995; 56:144.
Chiarian-Siteni V, Bononi A, Fomasa CV, Soraru M, Alaibao M, Ferrazzi E, Redelutti R, Paserico A, Monfardini S, Salvagno L. Phase II trial of interferon-α-2a plus psoralen with ultraviolet light A in patients with cutaneous T-cell-lymphoma. Cancer 2002; 95:569–575.
Kuzel TM, Roenigk HH, Samuelson E, Hermann JJ, Hurria A, Rademaker AW, Rosen ST. Effectiveness of interferon alfa-2a combined with phototherapy for mycosis fungoides and the Sezary syndrome. J Clin Oncol 1995; 13:257–263.
Mostow EN, Neckel SL, Oberhelman L, Anderson TF, Cooper KD. Complete remissions in psoralen and UV-A (PUVA) -refractory mycosis funoides-type cutaneous T-cell lymphoma with combined interferon alfa and PUVA. Arch Dermatol 1993; 129:747–752.
Rajan GP, Seifert B, Prümmer O, Joller-Jemelka HI, Burg G, Dummer R. Incidence and in-vivo relevance of anti-interferon antibodies during treatment of low-grade cutaneous T-cell lymphomas with interferon alpha-2a combined with acitretin or PUVA. Arch Dermatol Res 1996; 288:543–548.
Roenigk HH, Kuzel TM, Skoutelis AP, Springer E, Yu G, Caro W, Gilyon K, Variakojis D, Kaul K, Bunn PA, Evans L, Rosen ST. Photochemotherapy alone or combined with interferon alpha-2a in the treat-

ment of cutaneous T-cell lymphoma, J Invest Dermatol 1990; 95:198S–205S.

Stadler R, Otte HG, Luger T, Henz BM, Kühl P, Zwingers T, Sterry W. Prospective randomized multicenter clinical trial on the use of interferon α-2a plus acitretin versus interferon α-2a plus PUVA in patients with cutaneous T-cell lymphoma stages I and II. Blood 1998; 92:3578–3581.

Combination Therapy—Nitrogen Mustard

Price NM, Constantine VS, Hoppe RT, Fuks ZY, Farber EM. Topical mechlorethamine therapy for mycosis fungoides. Br J Dermatol 1977; 97:547–550.

Monk BE, Vollum DI, duVivier AWP. Combination topical nitrogen mustard and photochemotherapy for mycosis fungoides. Clin Exp Dermatol 1984; 9:243–247.

Du Vivier A, Vollum DI. Photochemotherapy and topical nitrogen mustard in the treatment of mycosis fungoides. Br J Dermatol 1980; 102:319–322.

Combination Therapy—Bexarotene

McGinnis KS, Shapiro M, Vittorio CC, Rook AH, Junkins-Hopkins JM. Psoralen plus long-wave UV-A (PUVA) and bexarotene therapy. Arch Dermatolatol 2003; 139:771–775.

Singh F, Lebwohl MG. Cutaneous T-cell lymphoma treatment using bexarotene and PUVA: a case series. J Am Acad Dermatol 2004; 51:570–573.

Photosensitivity

Molin L, Volden G. Treatment of light-sensitive mycosis fungoides with PUVA and prednisone. Photodermatology 1987; 4:106–107.

Volden G, Thune PO. Light sensitivity in mycosis fungoides. Br J Dermatol 1977; 97:279–284.

17

Vitiligo

INTRODUCTION

Many physicians are fatalistic regarding the treatment of vitiligo and either actively discourage patients from seeking therapy or tell them they should just live with their disease. In part this attitude is due to a belief that vitiligo is "just a cosmetic problem." This viewpoint ignores the profound psychological and social disturbances that vitiligo can cause in patients with dark skin and patients who tan well during summer. Furthermore, using this reasoning many dermatologic complaints can be similarly classified as only cosmetic in nature. Another reason for fatalism is the belief that treatment is almost always unsuccessful. This belief is wrong. UV therapy, which is the most effective means of achieving repigmentation, but is not the only treatment, is less effective in vitiligo than it is in psoriasis, and yet many patients achieve a satisfactory result.

A positive approach to the management of vitiligo requires an initial detailed consultation to assess the disease and the effect it has on the patient, followed by an explanation of the nature of the disease process and the likely prognosis, the treatment options available, what UV therapy will involve if this option is taken, and the expected therapeutic result. If a tentative decision to begin UV therapy is made, a good approach is to suggest that the final decision be delayed until the next visit so the patient has time to consider all the information provided.

Finally, an important point to keep in mind when evaluating a study of repigmentation of vitiligo by a new agent: these studies have little relationship to the real world. Most studies evaluate the percentage of repigmentation as their end point. However, if a given macule of vitiligo is totally filled in, the pigment is usually retained, but if it is only partially repigmented, the pigment is usually lost over the next 6–12 months. Obviously, for patients, partial repigmentation may be a wasted effort.

TREATMENT OPTIONS

Each of the treatment options should be explained, starting with simplest and progressing through more complicated treatments. A handout summarizing these options is very useful to educate patients. Finally, since there is no uniformly effective treatment for vitiligo, "snake oil" treatments are not uncommon and patients should be warned to check with their physician before using any new treatment.

Protection

The avoidance of sun exposure and lifetime use of an effective sunscreen on vitiligo at exposed sites is the minimal treatment that must be offered to any patient in order to avoid actinic damage and skin cancer.

Reduction of Contrast

Use of a broad-spectrum sunscreen on both normal and depigmented skin plus avoidance of sun exposure will make vitiligo less obvious by preventing tanning of normal skin. This is often the best option in patients with fair skin.

Cosmetic Concealment

The areas of vitiligo can be masked with Covermark®, Dermablend®, or other similar products. This is a suitable approach for patients with small areas of vitiligo on the face who do not want to undergo a course of PUVA therapy. Liquid dyes such as Vitadye® are also available, but they seldom provide a suitable match for skin color, and in dark-skinned patients a greenish hue often results. Self-tanning lotions containing dihydroxyacetone are another approach and the effect lasts several days; the degree of concealment decreases with increasing skin type.

Repigmentation

There are several modalities shown to be able to restore pigmentation in vitiligo (Table 1).

Table 1 Agents Producing Repigmentation in Vitiligo

UV therapy
Narrowband UVB phototherapy
Oral PUVA therapy
Topical PUVA therapy
Excimer laser
Topical corticosteroids
Immunomodulators
Tacrolimus
Pimecrolimus
Calcipotriene
Melanocyte grafts

UV Therapy

Some form of UV therapy is the safest and most effective means of producing repigmentation. Narrowband UVB phototherapy is being used more but oral PUVA therapy remains the gold standard as it is more effective. Topical PUVA therapy is used for localized disease in some centers but unexpected blistering phototoxic reactions are a frequent problem. The excimer laser has been used in some studies but this is a very expensive and nonreimbursed treatment.

Topical Corticosteroids

Class I steroid creams and ointments do produce repigmentation but when used as monotherapy the dose required closely approaches or exceeds that required to produce striae. Less potent steroids are not as effective as monotherapy.

Immunomodulators

Tacrolimus and pimecrolimus can produce some repigmentation in vitiligo, and these agents do not produce atrophy. However, they should not be used in combination with UV therapy until their potential for promoting skin cancer has been evaluated.

Calcipotriene

When used as a monotherapy, calcipotriene can produce some repigmentation but its chief value is probably in combination with UV therapy.

Melanocyte Grafts

Various techniques have been used to transfer autologous melanocytes to areas of vitiligo and these will be discussed later.

Depigmentation

The pigmentation present in normal skin can be removed with the use of monobenzylether of hydroquinone (Benoquin®, Valeant Pharmaceuticals, Costa Mesa, CA). The result is that the patient is white in all areas that are exposed or over the whole body, depending on how large an area is treated. This is an option to be considered in patients with very extensive vitiligo and must be combined with a life-time program of avoidance of sun exposure and use of sunscreens. The process of depigmentation takes months to complete and the main adverse effect is that Benoquin® can cause an allergic contact dermatitis and if sensitized this precludes further use of the compound, possibly leaving partial depigmentation. For this reason, only limited areas of 2–5% of body surface should be treated.

SELECTION OF PATIENTS FOR UV THERAPY

There are four important points to consider before suggesting the use of UV therapy.

Site of Disease

Response to treatment varies greatly with different body sites (Table 2). Lesions on the face usually respond very well. The exceptions are total periorbital and perioral involvement, which usually give a poor response. The trunk and proximal limbs respond less well than the face but usually give a satisfactory result. The dorsa of the hands and feet are slow-responding areas, while the distal fingers and genitalia rarely, if ever, respond. In addition, segmental vitiligo at any site is often unresponsive to PUVA therapy.

Motivation of Patient

UV therapy for vitiligo is time-consuming and inconvenient so that unless the patient is strongly motivated, compliance will be poor and the results

Table 2   Response to UV by Site of Disease

Very responsive
  Face except total perioral and periorbital
Moderate response
  Trunk and proximal limbs
Slow response
  Dorsal hands and feet
No response
  Distal fingers
  Genitalia

---

unsatisfactory. The assumption that the prescribed therapy will be used because a patient has sought treatment is often wrong in the case of vitiligo. People with dark skin and young people are much more likely to adhere to treatment than fair-skinned or elderly patients. A problem that arises in patients with skin types II through IV is that the cosmetic disability is initially accentuated by PUVA therapy. Stimulation of a maximal pigmentary response of normal skin by therapy heightens the contrast with the vitiliginous skin. Patients must be warned that this will happen and will remain a problem until repigmentation of the macules occurs.

Age of Patient

This factor applies mainly to young children who are brought for treatment by concerned parents. For several reasons reassurance and an explanation are all that should be given. First, young children are usually not concerned with the vitiligo, and have a busy enough time growing up without indulging in a very time-consuming therapy. Second, there is no strong evidence that vitiligo of long duration responds differently from disease of recent onset, so there is probably nothing lost in waiting until the disease is a cosmetic problem for the child. Finally, a superior treatment may have been found by the time the child wants to be treated, which in girls is around 10–12 years of age and in boys is 14–16 years of age. An explanation along these lines is usually enough to quell the enthusiasm of most parents.

Extent of the Disease

This is the least important consideration except at the extremes. If a person has only a small area of vitiligo on covered skin, UV treatment is not indicated. Similarly, if vitiligo covers most of the body surface, treatment probably should be depigmentation or no treatment. However, between these two extremes there is a lot of uncertainty since some patients with extensive disease will show an excellent response and some with limited disease will respond poorly. The best approach is often to suggest a trial of 30 treatments and if there is no good repigmentation occurring by that time, treatment can be stopped.

INVESTIGATIONS

There is a significant association between vitiligo and thyroid disease, and as many as 20% of patients have abnormalities of thyroid function. Therefore, if there is any suggestion of such disease by history or physical examination, thyroid function tests should be ordered. Other endocrine abnormalities are not significantly associated with vitiligo.

Table 3 Choice of Treatment

Advantages of narrowband UVB therapy
   No need for pre- and posttreatment eye protection
   Avoids systemic medication
   Possibly less carcinogenic
Advantages of oral PUVA therapy
   Less frequent treatment (B.I.W. vs. T.I.W.)
   Probably more effective
   Carcinogenic risk is known

UV THERAPY

Choice of Treatment

The choice of treatment usually is between narrowband UVB phototherapy and oral PUVA therapy and the advantages of each treatment are outlined in Table 3. Topical PUVA therapy is usually not considered because the response rate is low and phototoxic reactions are common. Oral PUVA therapy is considered superior to narrowband phototherapy since a significant number of patients unresponsive to the latter subsequently respond to PUVA therapy, whereas the reverse situation has not been observed. However, in younger patients, narrowband UVB phototherapy is certainly the first choice for treatment.

Protocols

The protocols for treatment are outlined in Table 4. Patients are treated as skin type I and the dose of UV radiation is increased until a light pink color is induced in the vitiligo lesions and further increases are only made to maintain this degree of mild phototoxicity. Symptomatic erythema must be avoided as much as possible because marked phototoxicity may produce a Koebner

Table 4 Treatment protocols

Narrowband UVB therapy
   Starting dose: $300\,\mathrm{mJ/cm^2}$
   Increments: $10\text{–}15\%/\mathrm{Tx}$
   Frequency: T.I.W.
Oral PUVA therapy
   Methoxsalen dose: $0.4\,\mathrm{mg/kg}$
   Starting UVA dose: $1.5\,\mathrm{J/cm^2}$
   Increments: $0.5\,\mathrm{J/cm^2}$
   Frequency: B.I.W.

phenomenon and actually prevent improvement. Thus, in vitiligo it is necessary to follow a narrow line between minimal phototoxicity, which gives maximal response, and marked phototoxicity, which prevents a response.

When there is significant disease on the limbs an extra dose of UV radiation will be required for this area to produce a similar degree of phototoxicity as that produced on the face and torso. The starting dose and increments for this extra treatment are the same as the whole-body treatment. Similar considerations apply to disease on the hands and feet and a second extra treatment may be used for these sites.

When disease is limited, as, for example, with involvement restricted to the face, exposure is restricted to that area but it must be explained to the patient that clothing has to be standard for every treatment.

Response to Treatment

Improvement of disease on UV therapy usually consists of the development of perifollicular dots of pigmentation in the areas of vitiligo. These dots gradually enlarge and coalesce to produce even pigmentation of the whole area. Less often the repigmentation occurs from the margins with a hyperpigmented border of macules or patches and their progressive shrinkage in size. Occasionally, in people with skin types IV–VI, new pigmentation will be darker than in normal skin, but this is not a problem since the pigmentation will become even when treatment is stopped. When repigmentation of a macule is complete, the pigment is usually retained without further treatment but there are recurrences in a few patients. In addition, new areas of vitiligo may appear during treatment, but in this situation treatments should be continued because complete repigmentation may occur.

Response to treatment is slow and depends on the location of the disease. Dots of pigment should be seen within 25 exposures with facial lesions, and 50 exposures with disease elsewhere; if not, treatment should be stopped. Complete repigmentation usually requires 50–300 exposures. While about 70% of patients achieve satisfactory improvement, only a few patients achieve complete repigmentation of all macules if areas other than the face are involved.

Adjunctive Treatment

The results of UV therapy can be improved by three forms of adjunctive therapy.

Topical Corticosteroids

Potent topical corticosteroids produce repigmentation in vitiligo but the difference between a therapeutic dose and that which produces striae is very small, so that striae are an almost inevitable consequence of treatment. However, corticosteroids used moderately at sites unlikely to be affected by atrophy can usefully potentiate the effect of UV therapy. The dorsa of the hands and feet, both of which are poorly responding areas, can often be greatly helped by concomitant use of fluocinonide 0.05% cream applied daily in addition to UV therapy. Repigmentation induced by use of corticosteroids often occurs as a uniform return of pigment across the whole macule or patch.

Topical Calcipotriene

Twice daily application of calcipotriene cream or ointment can produce repigmentation in vitiligo and there is some evidence that it can enhance the effect of UV therapy although the results of studies have not been consistent. Therefore, it can be a useful additive treatment for areas that are slow to respond.

Melanocyte Grafts

The concept of transferring melanocytes into areas of vitiligo is an attractive one, particularly in combination with UV therapy so that nonresponding areas can be treated in patients who have stable disease. The idea is to sprinkle melanocytes in these areas and then use exposure to UV therapy to expand the grafts and produce even repigmentation. The idea does have some drawbacks, and the main one in the United States is that there is no reimbursement for the surgical procedure. Several procedures have been used to harvest melanocytes.

Epidermal grafts: The epidermis is removed from the buttock using a suction-blister machine and transferred to the recipient site, which has been prepared by removing the epidermis by freezing or laser ablation. The procedure is tedious and time consuming but the results are very satisfactory.

Punch biopsy grafts: This approach has the disadvantage of giving a pebbly uneven surface in the area of vitiligo and scars in the donor site.

In vitro culture of melanocytes: Melanocytes can be harvested from normal skin removed by a shave biopsy, grown in culture, and then injected into areas of vitiligo. This technique requires access to a specialized laboratory, has a risk that cells might transform in culture, and is not suitable for combining with subsequent exposure to UV therapy.

OTHER DISORDERS OF PIGMENTATION

Postinflammatory hypopigmentation may respond to UV therapy. The most common example is the so-called pityriasis alba, which may be an end result of eczema and is particularly common in patients with skin types IV–VI. This condition usually responds rapidly in 10–20 treatments, and there is no necessity for prolonged maintenance treatment.

Patients with piebaldism who have functional melanocytes might be expected to respond to PUVA therapy, but this has not occurred in the few patients treated. PUVA therapy is contraindicated in albinism, because the risk of skin cancer is great and the theoretical benefits are very uncertain.

BIBLIOGRAPHY

PUVA Therapy

Grimes PE, Minus JR, Chakrabarti SG, Enterline J, Halder R, Gough E, Kenney JA. Determination of optimal photochemotherapy for vitiligo. J Am Acad Dermatol 1982; 7:771–778.

Lassus A, Halme K, Eskelinen A, Ranki A, Puska P, Salo O. Treatment of vitiligo with oral methoxsalen and UVA. Photodermatology 1984; 1:170–173.

Ortel B, Maytum DJ, Gange RW. Long persistence of monofunctional 8-methoxypsoralen-DNA adducts in human skin in vivo. Photochem Photobiol 1991; 54:645–650.

Ortel B, Gange RW. An action spectrum for the elicitation of erythema in skin persistently sensitized by photobound 8-methoxypsoralen. J Invest Dermatol 1990; 94:781–785.

Parrish JA, Fitzpatrick TB, Shea C, Pathak MA. Photochemotherapy of vitiligo. Arch Dermatol 1976; 112:1531–1534.

Ortonne JP, Macdonald DM, Micoud A, Thivolet J. PUVA-induced repigmentation of vitiligo: a histochemical (split-DOPA) and ultrastructural study. Br J Dermatol 1979; 101:1–7.

Skouge J, Morison WL. Vitiligo treatment with a combination of PUVA therapy and epidermal autografts. Arch Dermatol 1995; 131: 1257–1258.

Narrowband UVB Phototherapy

Dogra S, Parsad D. Combination of narrowband UV-B and topical calcipotriene in vitiligo. Arch Dermatol 2003; 139:393.

Kullavanijaya P, Lim HW. Topical calcipotriene and narrowband ultraviolet B in the treatment of vitiligo. Photodermatol Photoimmunol Photomed 2004; 20:248–251.

Natta R, Somsak T, Wisuttida T, Laor L. Narrowband ultraviolet B radiation therapy for recalcitrant vitiligo in Asians. J Am Acad Dermatol 2003; 49:473–476.

Njoo MD, Bos JD, Westerhof W. Treatment of generalized vitiligo in children with narrow-band (TL-01) UVB radiation therapy. J Am Acad Dermatol 2000; 42:245–253.

Scherschun L, Kim JJ, Lim HW. Narrow-band ultraviolet B is a useful and well-tolerated treatment for vitiligo. J Am Acad Dermatol 2001; 44:999–1003.

Vazquez-Lopez F, Claveria J. Calcipotriene and vitiligo. Arch Dermatol 2003; 139:1656–1657.

Westerhof W, Nieuweboer-Krobotova L. Treatment of vitiligo with UV-B radiation vs topical psoralen plus UV-A. Arch Dermatol 1997; 133:1525–1528.

Yashar SS, Gielczyk R, Scherschun L, Lim HW. Narrow-band ultraviolet B treatment for vitiligo, pruritus, and inflamatory dermatoses. Photodermatol Photoimmunol Photomed 2003; 19:164–168.

18

Photodermatoses

INTRODUCTION

Photosensitivity can be reduced or eliminated in patients with certain photo-dermatoses by deliberate exposure to PUVA therapy, UVB phototherapy, or other wavebands of radiation (Table 1). This therapy is called desensitization and is the treatment of choice in many severely incapacitated patients. The management of some conditions, such as PMLE, is easy and routine so that it can be safely performed in any office. In contrast, management of solar urticaria and chronic photosensitive eczemas is not easy since it requires phototesting and close monitoring of patients.

The mechanism of desensitization is unknown; its use arose from the observation that many patients with PMLE "harden" or lose their photo-sensitivity as summer progresses. This was assumed to be due to the protective effect of sun-induced tanning and epidermal hyperplasia. The protective effect is local in the skin because areas shielded during desensitization remain photosensitive. However, PUVA therapy for photosensitive eczema can reduce photosensitivity by more than a factor of 40, and this cannot be explained simply on the basis of skin protection. Presumably, some basic mechanism responsible for triggering the disease is inactivated by the treatment.

Table 1 Photodermatoses Responsive to UV Therapy

Polymorphous light eruption
Solar urticaria
Chronic photosensitive eczema
   Chronic actinic dermatitis
   Actinic prurigo
   Photoexacerbated atopic eczema
Erythropoietic protoporphyria

POLYMORPHOUS LIGHT ERUPTION

PMLE is the most common photodermatosis and afflicts 12–21% of the population. There is a wide range in the degree of photosensitivity, and the vast majority of patients have mild disease resulting in minimal interference with normal outdoor activity. These people seldom consult a physician and instead learn to avoid a threshold dose of sunlight.

Diagnosis and Evaluation

The diagnosis and evaluation of PMLE is simple and straightforward (Table 2). The diagnosis is readily made from the history of a papular or papulovesicular eruption that begins hours or a day or so after a specific exposure to sunlight and lasts from days to a week or more. An idea of whether it is induced by UVA or UVB radiation can be determined by asking whether the rash can occur behind glass as in a car or after application of a sunscreen. Positive answers to these questions usually indicate that UVA radiation is the eliciting waveband, and, conversely, negative answers point to UVB radiation.

    The next step is to evaluate the severity of the condition in terms of how much inconvenience and morbidity it causes. Obviously, this evaluation is very subjective and varies with the individual but it will decide further evaluation and management. PMLE triggered by all-day exposure to sunlight in the tropics is mild disease, requires no further evaluation, and can be managed by advice to avoid a threshold exposure and application of a

Table 2 Diagnosis and Evaluation of PMLE

History
Eliciting waveband
   UVB or UVA
Severity
   Mild, moderate, or severe
See the rash, do a biopsy and a lupus package

broad-spectrum sunscreen. PMLE triggered by a 15 min exposure to the sun in spring in Baltimore is severe disease and requires further evaluation and consideration of desensitization with a course of UV therapy. The next steps in the evaluation of moderate and severe cases are

- *See the rash.* Sunlight produced the rash and thus is the most reliable radiation source to reproduce it. The patient is instructed to expose the affected area to sunlight and return when the rash has developed.
- *Do a biopsy.* The histologic findings in PMLE are not diagnostic, but this step is helpful in eliminating LE, which is the most important alternative diagnosis.
- *Do a lupus package on serum.* This step is essential if there is any suggestion of a diagnosis of LE or if UV therapy is being considered.

Management

Protocols

Various protocols for prophylactic treatment have been published but the ones outlined in Table 3 give satisfactory results. Once the course of treatment is completed, the patient must have a 1 hr exposure to sunlight around midday each week to maintain protection, or if this is not possible, a once weekly maintenance treatment.

Timing

Treatment is given in spring for patients who have problems during most of the summer months. For patients visiting a sunny climate such as a winter vacation in Hawaii, the course of treatment can be given immediately before departure.

Problems

About half the patients will develop PMLE during the course of treatment and this can be managed by application of a potent topical corticosteroid or, if severe and extensive, a brief course of prednisone while treatment is continued.

Table 3 Prophylactic UV Therapy of PMLE

Narrowband UVB therapy three times a week for 5 weeks
Oral PUVA therapy three times a week for 4 weeks
Broadband UVB therapy five times a week for 3 weeks

Results

Narrowband UVB phototherapy and PUVA therapy give similar results with 80–90% of patients being completely or almost completely protected. Patients not protected are usually those with the lowest threshold for disease and the options are to use a longer course or switch to the other waveband. Broadband UVB therapy is less effective and protects 60–70% of patients.

SOLAR URTICARIA

Solar urticaria is much less common than PMLE but causes marked disability since the patients are often very photosensitive.

Diagnosis and Evaluation

The history usually provides the diagnosis when the patient recounts a sudden onset of pruritus, redness, and hives within minutes of exposure to sunlight, and these symptoms persist for an hour or so. The main disorder to consider in the differential diagnosis is erythropoietic protoporphyria, which can be excluded by fluorescent microscopic examination of a blood smear. The rash can be easily produced, and this is best done as part of a determination of the action spectrum by exposure to broadband sources of UVB, UVA, and visible radiation. Use of incremental doses of the eliciting waveband(s) provides a measurement of the minimum urtication dose (MUD).

Management

The management of solar urticaria is usually difficult. Sunscreens are of little value because of the degree of photosensitivity and most patients are sensitive to UVA or visible radiation. Antihistamines are of benefit in a few patients. A trial of terfenadine in a dose of 60–120 mg twice daily is worthwhile. Prednisone is usually without effect. Desensitization by exposure to radiation has been successful in a few limited trials and is the treatment of choice in severely incapacitated patients. Several approaches have been used.

Oral Puva Therapy

Patients who are not sensitive to UVA radiation are given a course of therapy using a regular T.I.W. schedule. Patients who are sensitive to UVA radiation are started at 80% of their MUD, and the dose is increased 0.5 J/cm^2 each treatment on a T.I.W. schedule. If urticaria occurs, the dose is held constant until this reaction ceases. The patients are asked to expose themselves to sunlight once a week, and PUVA therapy is continued until they are able to tolerate 1 or 2 hr or more of exposure around noon without developing urticaria. It usually requires 4–6 weeks of treatment to reach this point, and thereafter the patients are instructed to have a 1 hr exposure to sunlight three times each week during the summer. This treatment achieves tolerance of at least 2 hr of sun exposure in most patients, and a few are able to tolerate all-day exposure. There is no evidence that this treatment produces remission of disease so the course of therapy has to be repeated each spring.

Phototherapy

Narrowband UVB therapy: One patient with solar urticaria induced by visible light was successfully treated with T.I.W. treatment for 5 weeks and was able to tolerate 3 hr of sunlight exposure without symptoms.

UVA phototherapy: UVA phototherapy, without psoralen, using the same doses of radiation as in PUVA therapy of solar urticaria, is effective in desensitizing some patients who are sensitive to UVA radiation. It is unclear whether this treatment is effective in patients who are sensitive to other wavebands. However, it is intriguing that in these case reports, treatment with UVA alone did result in increased tolerance to sunlight. Clearly, this treatment requires further evaluation.

Exposure to eliciting waveband: Another approach is to deliberately expose patients to the eliciting waveband in doses sufficient to produce urticaria and repeat this at hourly intervals until the skin is nonreactive; the tolerance is then maintained by daily exposure. Due to the risk of systemic effects, only one area can be treated at a time, so it takes a week or more to achieve total-body tolerance. The patient then requires a home phototherapy unit to maintain the desensitized state.

CHRONIC PHOTOSENSITIVE ECZEMA

Three conditions can be grouped, at least from a therapeutic standpoint, under the collective term of chronic photosensitive eczema, since they all respond to the same treatments: chronic actinic dermatitis (CAD), actinic prurigo, and photoexacerbated atopic eczema. These patients present with an eczematous eruption that is most marked on exposed areas and is often present year round but is usually worse in summer.

Diagnosis and Evaluation

The skin biopsy and detection of a low MED to one or more wavebands on phototesting (Table 4) will confirm the diagnosis of a photosensitive eczema. The sites of lowered erythermal responses will usually become eczematous within a week. Photopatch testing is required in patients with CAD. Patients with CAD tend to be older, frequently have multiple medical problems, and

Table 4 Evaluation of Chronic Photosensitive Eczema

Skin biopsy
Phototesting
   UVB, UVA, and visible light
Determination of minimum eliciting dose
Photopatch testing
General medical assessment

since suppression of photosensitivity with prednisone is probably required, consultation with an internist is advised.

Management

Three treatments have been used successfully in this condition: cyclosporin, azathioprin, and UV desensitization but only the latter will be discussed here. The main advantage of desensitization over the other two treatments is that if the patient can be cleared and maintained in a clear state, long-term remission is likely to occur.

PUVA Desensitization

Most of these patients are exquisitely photosensitive and the action spectrum for their eruption includes UVA radiation. Thus, PUVA therapy cannot be used alone but must be combined with agents to suppress the photosensitivity. In the past these patients were admitted to hospital for a couple of weeks and PUVA desensitization was done using large doses of prednisone for suppression but this is not possible today. An alternative outpatient regimen is now used combining prednisone and mycophenolate mofetil (Cellcept®, Roche); this is outlined in Table 5. A blood count and biochemical screen is required before starting this regimen and a weekly blood count is required while on mycophenolate due to a risk of neutropenia. The starting dose of UVA radiation is according to skin type with the usual increases up to a maximal dose suitable for the skin type. Long-term maintenance at a frequency of Q.W. during summer and Q2W during winter

Table 5 PUVA Desensitization of Chronic Photosensitive Eczema

Commence mycophenolate mofetil in dose of 1 g twice daily
Three weeks later: start prednisone 40 mg daily
Following day: start oral PUVA T.I.W.
Two weeks later: start tapering prednisone over the next 2 weeks
Stop mycophenolate 4 weeks after stopping prednisone and reduce PUVA therapy to
   QW treatment

is required. A spontaneous remission eventually occurs but this can take 2–7 years.

Narrowband UVB Phototherapy

Actinic prurigo has been treated with this modality as a monotherapy TIW for 5 weeks with a good result although the rash was initially exacerbated in most patients.

ERYTHROPOIETIC PROTOPORPHYRIA

There are case reports of the successful use of PUVA therapy and narrowband UVB therapy as prophylactic treatment to suppress photosensitivity in this rare condition. These reports have documented increased tolerance to UVA and visible light. I have treated one patient with oral PUVA therapy (TIW for 4 weeks) in spring and she was able to tolerate more than 3 hr of sunlight during summer without any symptoms.

BIBLIOGRAPHY

Polymorphous Light Eruption

Addo HA, Sharma SC. UVB phototherapy and photochemotherapy (PUVA) in the treatment of polymorphic light eruption and solar urticaria. Br J Dermatol 1987; 116:539–547.

Bilsand D, George SA, Gibbs NK, Aitchison T, Johnson BE, Ferguson J. A comparison of narrow band phototherapy (TL-01) and photochemotherapy (PUVA) in the management of polymorphic light eruption. Br J Dermatol 1993; 129:708–712.

Gschnait F, Hönigsmann H, Brenner W, Fritsch P, Wolff K. Induction of UV light tolerance by PUVA in patients with polymorphous light eruption. Br J Dermatol 1978; 99:293–296.

Gschnait F, Schwarz T, Ladich I. Treatment of polymorphous light eruption. Arch Dermatol Res 1983; 275:379–382.

Jansen CT, Karvonen J, Malmiharju T. PUVA therapy for polymorphous light eruptions: comparison of systemic methoxsalen and topical trioxsalen regimens and evaluation of local protective mechanisms. Acta Dermatol 1982; 62:317–320.

Ling TC, Gibbs NK, Rhodes LE. Treatment of polymorphic light eruption. Photodermatol Photoimmunol Photomed 2003; 19:217–227.

Man I, Dawe RS, Ferguson J. Artificial hardening for polymorphic light eruption: practical points from ten years' experience. Photodermatol Photoimmunol Photomed 1999; 15:96–99.

Molin L, Volden G. Treatment of polymorphous light eruption with PUVA and prednisone. Photodermatology 1987; 4:107–108.

Morison WL, Momtaz TK, Mosher DB. UV-B phototherapy in the prophylaxis of polymorphous light eruption. Br J Dermatol 1982; 106:231–233.

Murphy GM, Logan RA, Lovell CR, Morris RW, Hawk JLM, Magnus IA. Prophylactic PUVA and UVB therapy in polymorphic light eruption—a controlled trial. Br J Dermatol 1987; 116:531–538.

Palmer RA, Friedmann PS. A comparison of six and 12 PUVA treatments in the prophylaxis of polymorphic light eruption. Clin Exp Dermatol 2004; 29:141–143.

Parrish JA, LeVine MJ, Morison WL, Gonzalez E, Fitzpatrick TB. Comparison of PUVA and beta-carotene in the treatment of polymorphous light eruption. Br J Dermatol 1978; 100:187–191.

Rücker BU, Häberle M, Koch HU, Bocionek P, Schriever K-H, Hornstein OP. Ultraviolet light hardening in polymorphous light eruption-a controlled study comparing different emission spectra. Photodermatol Photoimmunol Photomed 1991; 8:73–78.

Solar Urticaria

Bernhard JD, Jaenicke K, Momtaz TK, Parrish JA. Ultraviolet A phototherapy in the prophylaxis of solar urticaria. J Am Acad Dermatol 1984; 10:29–33.

Beissert S, Ständer H, Schwarz T. UVA rush hardening for the treatment of solar urticaria. J Am Acad Dermatol 2000; 42:1030–1032.

Collins P, Ferguson J. Narrow-band UVB (TL-01) phototherapy: an effective preventative treatment for the photodermatoses. Br J Dermatol 1995; 132:956–963.

Dawe RS, Ferguson J. Prolonged benefit following ultraviolet A phototherapy for solar urticaria. Br J Dermatol 1997; 137:144–148.

Holzdena E, Hoffman A, Plewig G. PUVA-treatment for solar urticaria and persistent light reaction. Arch Dermatol Res 1980; 269:87–91.

Hudson-Peacock MJ, Farr PM, Diffey BL, Goodship THJ. Combined treatment of solar urticaria with plasmapheresis and PUVA. Br J Dermatol 1993; 128:440–442.

Keahey TM, Lavker RM, Kaidbey KH, Atkins PC, Zweiman B. Studies on the mechanism of clinical tolerance in solar urticaria. Br J Dermatol 1984; 110:327–338.

Parrish JA, Jaenicke KF, Morison WL, Momtaz K, Shea C. Solar urticaria: treatment with PUVA and mediator inhibitors. Br J Dermatol 1982; 106:575–580.

Ramsay CA. Solar urticaria treatment by inducing tolerance to artificial radiation and natural light. Arch Dermatol 1977; 113:1222–1225.

Chronic Photosensitive Eczema

Farr PM, Diffey BL. Treatment of actinic prurigo with PUVA: mechanism of action. Br J Dermatol 1989; 120:411–418.

Hunziker T, Krebs KA. Orale photochemotherapie bei aktinischem retikuloid. Dermatologica 1982; 165:114–122.

Lindberg L, Larko O, Roupe G. Successful PUVA-treatment for musk ambrette-induced persistent light reaction. Photodermatology 1986; 3:111–112.

Morison WL. Chronic photosensitivity. Dermatol Clin 1986; 4:261–266.

Morison WL, White HAD, Gonzalez E, Parrish JA, Fitzpatrick TB. Oral methoxsalen photochemotherapy of uncommon photodermatoses. Acta Dermatol 1979; 59:366–368.

Nousari HC, Anhalt GJ, Morison WL. Mycophenolate in psoralen-UV-A desensitization therapy for chronic actinic dermatitis. Arch Dermatol 1999; 135:1128–1129.

Erythropoietic Protoporphyria

Collins P, Ferguson J. Narrow-band UVB (TL-01) phototherapy: an effective preventative treatment for the photodermatoses. Br J Dermatol 1995; 132:956–963.

Ros A. PUVA therapy for erythropoietic protoporphyria. Photodermatology 1988; 5:148–149.

19

Miscellaneous Diseases

INTRODUCTION

In addition to the diseases of the skin that have already been discussed, there are at least 40 other conditions reported to respond to PUVA therapy or UV phototherapy. Many of these conditions are rare and experience is limited to case reports, but some have been studied in controlled or open trials (Table 1). For ease of reference, these diseases will be discussed alphabetically.

ALOPECIA AREATA

Several studies have evaluated PUVA therapy in the various forms of alopecia areata. There are some differences in the results but a consensus, including our own experience, is as follows:

- Circumscribed alopecia of the scalp responds better than totalis, which in turn responds better than universalis.
- Whole-body exposure, even for local disease, yields better results than local exposure of the scalp, but local treatment, as with topical PUVA therapy, can produce regrowth.
- If significant regrowth has not occurred by 30 treatments, improvement is unlikely to occur.
- Between 30% and 50% of totalis and universalis patients respond with cosmetically acceptable regrowth. More than half of these patients lose most of this hair if treatment is stopped. While

Table 1 Response of Various Dermatoses to UV Therapy

	Controlled trial	Open trial	Anecdote
Alopecia areata		++	
Amyloidosis			+++
Darier's disease			++
Dermatitis Herpetiformis		++	
Eosinophilic cellulitis			+++
Eosinophilic fasciitis			+++
Eosinophilis pustular folliculitis		+++	
Erythema multiforme			+++
Erythrokeratoderma			+++
Flegel's disease			++
Graft-versus-host disease	++		
Granuloma annulare		+++	
Granuloma faciale			+++
Histiocytosis X			+++
Hypereosinophilic syndrome			+++
Ichthyosis linearis circumflexa			++
Keratosis lichenoides chronica			+
Lichen planus	+++		
Lymphomatoid papulosis			++
Mastocytosis			
Urticaria pigmentosa	++		
Diffuse cutaneous		++	
Necrobiosis lipoidica		++	
Papuloerythroderma			+++
Perforating dermatosis		+++	
Pigmented purpuric dermatoses		+++	
Pityriasis lichenoides			
Acute		+++	
Chronic		+++	
Pityriasis rosea	+++		
Pityriasis rubra pilaris			++
Pruritis			
Renal failure	++		
Primary ciliary cirrhosis			++
Polycythemia vera		++	
HIV infection		++	
Idiopathic			++
Neurotic excoriations			+++

(Continued)

Table 1 Response of Various Dermatoses to UV Therapy (*Continued*)

	Controlled trial	Open trial	Anecdote
Sclerosing skin diseases			
Linea morphea		++	
Generalized morphea		++	
Systemic sclerosis			++
Lichen sclerosis			++
Sclerodema			++
Scleromyxodema			++
Lichen myxoedematosus			++
Subcorneal pustular dermatosis			+++
Transient acantholytic dermatosis			+++
Urticaria			
Idiopathic		++	
Dermographism		++	
Physical			++
Cholinergic			++
Schnitzler syndrome			+++
Vasculitis			++
Chilblains	−		
Male-pattern baldness	−		

Note: +++, complete response; ++, partial response; +, minimal response; −, no response.

long-term maintenance treatment can prevent this from occurring the risks of this approach must be evaluated in the individual patient.

Thus, PUVA therapy is not an ideal treatment for alopecia areata, but in the absence of any other successful therapy it is sometimes useful.

AMYLOIDOSIS

Lichen amyloidosis and macular amyloidosis are rarely seen in North America and Europe but are common diseases in Asia, the Middle East, Central, and South America. They are characterized by intensely pruritic and pigmented papules or macules on the forearms, legs, and the interscapular area. These conditions have been successfully treated with broadband UVB, topical PUVA, and oral PUVA. PUVA therapy is more effective than UVB and appears to produce a longer remission of at least 1 year or more. Two patients with macular amyloidosis that we treated had remission of pruritis after 20 treatments using a regular oral PUVA schedule; pigmentation merged with the PUVA-induced tan after 30 treatments and limited maintenance for 3 months was followed by a long-term remission.

DARIER'S DISEASE

Keratosis follicularis is usually considered to be a photoaggravated dermatosis but some patients have no history of exacerbation by sunlight. There is one case reported to respond to etretinate and oral PUVA therapy and I have treated an extensive exacerbation in one patient with oral PUVA therapy alone. This patient had no history of aggravation by sunlight and his exacerbation cleared in 35 treatments and his disease has remained quiescent for 8 years.

DERMATITIS HERPETIFORMIS

Five patients uncontrolled by dapsone and diet or intolerant of dapsone had a good response to PUVA therapy in terms of clearance of lesions and immunoreactants in the skin. The effect was short-lived, but maintenance treatment was successful.

EOSINOPHILIC CELLULITIS (WELLS' SYNDROME)

There is one well-documented case report of this condition responding to several courses of PUVA therapy and a direct effect of the treatment is suggested by a covered control site remaining unchanged. Long-term maintenance was required.

EOSINOPHILIC FASCIITIS

There is one case report of a patient treated with bath PUVA therapy with complete resolution by 50 treatments as judged clinically and by ultrasound.

EOSINOPHILIC PUSTULAR FOLLICULITIS

This condition occurs in association with HIV infection, usually in its end stage of AIDS with a low CD4 count, but it can rarely occur in otherwise healthy people. It presents with follicular pustules over the face, trunk, and extremities and an intense pruritus. One open trial found that UVB phototherapy relieved the pruritus rapidly and produced some clearance of the lesions; maintenance therapy was essential to prevent a return of the pruritis. PUVA therapy can produce complete clearance of lesions, and Q2W maintenance appears to be adequate.

ERYTHEMA MULTIFORME

The chronic form of this condition is rare but can result in significant morbidity. We treated a patient with a 2-year history of the disease on the palms and soles using oral PUVA therapy and local exposure of the hands and feet. After five treatments, the patient developed an extensive eruption of typical lesions of erythema multiforme over the trunk, face, hands, and lips. Whole-body exposure was then begun with rapid clearance of both new and old lesions by treatment 16. Maintenance therapy was given for a year and then stopped without recurrence.

ERYTHROKERATODERMA: SYMMETRICAL AND PROGRESSIVE

A short course of PUVA therapy can clear this condition, according to a case report and personal experience of one case.

FLEGEL'S DISEASE

Hyperkeratosis follicularis perstans is a rare condition with hyperkeratotic papules on the limbs, particularly the dorsum of the feet. Clearance of the condition with oral PUVA therapy is reported in one patient and the positive result is supported by first clearing one limb only. The remission lasted for 2 months. Narrowband and broadband UVB therapies were not effective.

GRAFT-VERSUS-HOST DISEASE

Graft-versus-host disease (GVH) disease is a very significant problem after bone marrow transplantation and may occur early as acute disease or later as a chronic lichenoid GVH or sclerodermoid GVH disease. PUVA therapy is now widely used in many centers for treatment of each of the forms of the disease, usually as part of a multiagent immunosuppressive regimen because the disease involves multiple organs and the effect of PUVA therapy is limited to the skin and mucous membranes. The schedule of treatment is the same as for other diseases, with the exception that the starting dose is for a skin type I individual since about 20% of patients are photosensitive. The response rate is about 70% with 40% having total clearance. Maintenance treatment should be given for 3 months to prevent recurrence. The end stage of chronic sclerodermoid GVH disease, where there is no cellular infiltrate in the skin, does not respond to PUVA therapy. There is some preliminary information that indicates similar results can be obtained using narrowband UVB phototherapy and this has the possibility of being a less carcinogenic treatment in these immunosuppressed patients.

UV therapy is also useful in treating oral GVH disease. For PUVA therapy, the usual dose of methoxsalen is ingested, then an hour later the diseased area is exposed to UVA radiation starting at 0.5 J/cm^2 with increases of 0.5 J/cm^2 as tolerated on a T.I.W. schedule. About 50% clear within a few weeks and almost all are improved. A UVA light used by dentists for curing amalgam is a suitable light source or a targeted high-intensity source can be used. Again narrowband UVB therapy is an alternative approach. The MED and MPD in the mouth are about double the readings obtained on the skin of the back, so erythema is seldom a problem.

GRANULOMA ANNULARE

The diffuse or generalized form of this disease responds to oral and topical PUVA therapy with most patients requiring 30–40 treatments to clear. However, some patients with very indurated lesions may take as many as 100 treatments to clear. Maintenance requirements are variable but at least 3 months of treatment on a reduced schedule should be given after clearance.

GRANULOMA FACIALE

Topical PUVA therapy has been used to clear this condition in 30 treatments with no recurrence over the next 6 months.

HISTIOCYTOSIS X

The skin lesions of this condition respond to both PUVA and UVB phototherapy. PUVA therapy is the preferred treatment because of its greater effectiveness and ease of maintenance, which is required to sustain a remission.

HYPEREOSINOPHILIC SYNDROME

This condition can rarely have skin lesions in the absence of systemic organ involvement and there is one case report of clearance of the lesions with oral PUVA therapy with a remission lasting 2 years.

ICHTHYOSIS LINEARIS CIRCUMFLEXA

Two cases of this condition have been reported to respond to topical PUVA therapy with clearance of the psoriasiform skin lesions. Maintenance treatment was required in both instances.

KERATOSIS LICHENOIDES CHRONICA

This rare condition has been reported to improve on oral PUVA, which has been our experience in one patient only to be followed by a relapse in a few months.

LICHEN PLANUS

Several studies including one bilateral-comparison study have reported clearance of widespread lichen planus with oral and bath PUVA therapy in most patients in 30–40 treatments and maintenance therapy is not required. Two points of caution: in a few patients the disease will exacerbate on treatment and treatment has to be stopped; residual pigmentation at the sites of lesion commonly occurs in skin types IV–VI and patients must be warned that this will occur and it may last for years. Oral lichen planus can also be treated with local irradiation of the oral mucosa and the response is rapid with clearance in less than 20 treatments (see GVH disease for details).

LYMPHOMATOID PAPULOSIS

Oral PUVA therapy is effective in this condition in that most patients are improved with fewer lesions lasting a shorter period of time and a few patients have a complete remission. There is no information on the effect of PUVA therapy on risk of malignant transformation.

MASTOCYTOSIS

Urticaria Pigmentosa

Several studies have demonstrated the effectiveness of PUVA therapy in relieving symptoms of pruritus and urtication in this condition. The pigmented lesions also resolve, but this occurs more slowly. The improvement is associated with a decreased histamine content in skin and a reduction of the number of mast cells in the papillary dermis. However, PUVA therapy only produces a remission lasting a few months, and long-term maintenance therapy at a frequency of Q2W is required in most cases.

Diffuse Cutaneous Mastocytosis

This condition can present as a generalized bullous eruption in neonates or infants and there are two reports of oral PUVA therapy producing sustained remissions.

NECROBIOSIS LIPOIDICA DIABETICORUM

Several studies have examined the effect of PUVA therapy on necrobiosis lipoidica diabeticorum and in most instances topical methoxsalen has been used for 30–50 treatments. Most patients improve with flattening of the lesions and some reduction in the area of plaques and in a few patients all evidence of disease activity clears. Pain, if present, remits within a few treatments and ulceration, present in up to 30% of patients, heals rapidly. Improvement can be sustained for years without further treatment. Thin lesions respond better and more completely than markedly indurated lesions and this is simply a function of depth of penetration of UVA radiation.

PAPULOERYTHRODERMA

This is an uncommon form of erythroderma with sheets of pruritic red-brown papules that spare the skin folds and associated hematologic changes of eosinophilia and neutropenia. Oral PUVA therapy is effective in producing a complete remission in most cases, although relapses can occur.

PERFORATING DERMATOSIS

Acquired perforating dermatosis occurs in chronic renal failure and/or diabetes with or without hemodialysis. It is associated with marked pruritus. Narrowband UVB phototherapy produced a complete remission in all five patients treated in 10–15 treatments and the remission lasted for 1–8 months.

PIGMENTED PURPURIC DERMATOSES

This is a group of disorders that are a pleasure to treat since the patients have usually been exposed to multiple treatments without effect, and a brief course of only 10–12 treatments of oral PUVA therapy gives complete clearance in all patients with no need for maintenance, and rare relapses. UVB phototherapy is usually not effective.

PITYRIASIS LICHENOIDES

Both the acute and chronic forms of this condition respond almost universally to UV therapy. In the acute form (PLEVA) PUVA therapy is preferable, particularly if the lesions have much substance, and the disease slowly clears over 30–50 treatments. Maintenance therapy is not required and most patients do not relapse. UVB phototherapy is preferable in the chronic form (PLC) and it usually clears in 20–30 treatments. Relapse is very common and can occur within months in the absence of maintenance treatment.

PITYRIASIS ROSEA

Most patients with pityriasis rosea do not require active treatment, but patients with extensive, symptomatic, or persistent disease can be readily cleared with a short erythemogenic course of broadband UVB phototherapy and maintenance is not required. Narrowband UVB phototherapy is also effective.

PITYRIASIS RUBRA PILARIS

PUVA therapy alone may improve this condition but does not produce clearance of disease. However, combined treatment of PUVA plus methotrexate does clear some patients over the course of 3–4 months, and only limited maintenance therapy is required.

PRURITUS

Pruritus of diverse etiologies has been found to respond to UV therapy. These include the following.

Renal Failure

Pruritus is a feature of chronic renal failure and occurs in up to 80% of patients. Pruritus may commence with institution of dialysis treatment, although intensive hemodialysis may also relieve pruritus. Apart from renal transplantation, the treatment of uremic pruritus has been unsatisfactory.

Broadband UVB phototherapy provides relief or a complete remission of uremic pruritus in most patients. Doses close to the erythema threshold are required, but it is not necessary to produce erythema. A B.I.W. or T.I.W. schedule usually produces relief within 6–10 treatments, and each course should involve 12–20 exposures. Remissions may last several months, but some patients require constant maintenance therapy. UVA phototherapy is also reported to be beneficial in uremic pruritus with initial doses of 6 J/cm^2 rising to around 20 J/cm^2, but this is not a universal finding. A useful approach in the few patients who do not respond to UVB phototherapy is to use a combination of UVA and UVB phototherapy. Occasionally, a patient fails to respond to any of these approaches and it is necessary to use PUVA therapy. Psoralen and its products are presumably removed by dialysis since there is no increase in photosensitivity.

Primary Biliary Cirrhosis

This condition is characterized by obstructive jaundice and severe pruritus. There are several anecdotal reports of relief of the pruritus with UV phototherapy. In all cases, relief occurred within a few exposures but was of short duration, and prolonged maintenance therapy was essential. Both UVB and UVA radiation have been used, but the reports favor UVB phototherapy. Cholestyramine is an alternative therapy and was used as maintenance treatment in one report.

Polycythemia Vera

Pruritus is a common symptom in this condition and it can also occur in the myelodysplastic syndrome. Frequently, it is aquagenic and the intense exacerbation from bathing can last for hours. Oral PUVA therapy is very effective in producing a remission in 10–20 treatments. The duration of the remission varies from weeks to months and if short, maintenance treatment is required. Narrowband UVB phototherapy is also effective but it appears that maintenance treatment is essential.

HIV Infection

Pruritus in the absence of any primary skin lesions is common in patients with advanced HIV infection but it can occur at any stage. Broadband UVB, narrowband UVB, and PUVA therapy are all effective in relieving the symptoms and maintenance therapy is required until a spontaneous remission occurs.

Chronic Idiopathic Pruritus

This is the commonest form of pruritus and it usually afflicts people over the age of 70 years and has no underlying disease association. PUVA therapy is usually the preferred treatment, producing relief within 20 treatments, and long-term maintenance is often essential.

Neurotic Excoriations

Patients presenting with extensive excoriations mixed with atrophic scars and no evidence of primary lesions usually complain of pruritus as being the primary symptom. These patients respond to oral PUVA therapy with remission of the pruritus in 10–20 treatments and healing of all lesions by about 30 treatments. A remission will often last months but eventual relapse is typical.

SCLEROSING SKIN DISEASES

There has been great interest in recent years in evaluating the efficacy of PUVA therapy in this group of diseases with numerous case series and reports. There are no controlled trials but there is overwhelming evidence from clinical evaluation, histologic confirmation, and 20 MHz ultrasound assessment that oral PUVA, bath PUVA, and topical PUVA can stop progression of these diseases and reverse some of the sclerotic changes in the majority of patients. If all evidence of inflammation is eliminated, the recurrence rate is low and if the disease does become active again it usually responds to further treatment.

There are two important points to note when treating these diseases. First, treat early to minimize regional deformity. For example, contractures around joints in linear morphea and fibrotic lesions in generalized morphea will soften with treatment but if these changes have occurred they cannot be totally reversed. Second, treat aggressively and eliminate all evidence of inflammation. The main reason why it is only the majority of patients who respond is probably because of inadequate or incomplete treatment.

Linear Morphea

The affected area, such as a limb or face alone is treated and the end point of treatment is loss of induration of the most recent erythematous lesions. This will require 40–80 treatments followed by maintenance treatment with decreasing frequency over 3 months.

Generalized Morphea

Treatment is usually whole-body exposure and 50–100 treatments are required. Hyperpigmentation usually occurs at the site of all active lesions and takes several months to fade. Again, a 3-month period of maintenance is given to ensure that the disease is inactive.

Systemic Sclerosis

Acral and other skin involvement will soften with treatment, sometimes improving joint mobility but unfortunately there is no clear end point in this condition. There is no effect on systemic symptoms.

Lichen Sclerosis et Atrophicus

Experience in treating this condition is limited but it appears to respond to brief courses of topical or oral PUVA after 20–40 treatments at both extragenital and genital sites. Relief of pruritus is the first sign of improvement.

Scleredema

Bath PUVA and cream PUVA therapy have been reported to greatly improve this condition. I have treated three as a bilateral comparison of oral PUVA vs. no treatment with marked improvement clinically and on histology in two of the patients after 65 and 80 treatments. The condition may spontaneously resolve, so an internal control is useful.

Scleromyxodema/Lichen Myxoedematosus

There are case reports of each of these two conditions responding to oral PUVA therapy with relief of pruritus and marked improvement. The circulating paraprotein was unchanged.

SUBACUTE PRURIGO

This condition is not well defined but probably includes "itchy red bump" disease and papular eruption in black men. The features of the disease are

- Males and females usually over 50 years of age
- Intense pruritus
- Papular or urticarial lesions over trunk and proximal limbs
- Pathology consistent with insect bite reaction or dermal hypersensitivity reaction.

The condition is fairly common and at any one time I am treating three or four patients. Oral PUVA is very effective in relieving the pruritus within 10 treatments and clearing the rash in 20–25 treatments. Remission usually lasts 6–12 months and it can be recurrent over years. Narrowband UVB phototherapy is less effective in clearing the rash and continuous maintenance is required since remissions are short.

SUBCORNEAL PUSTULAR DERMATOSIS

Most patients with this condition respond to dapsone but a few do not respond or do not tolerate this therapy. UV therapy offers a good alternative treatment and broadband UVB, narrowband UVB, and oral PUVA therapy are all reported to be effective. Recurrences are common and long-term maintenance may be required.

TRANSIENT ACANTHOLYTIC DERMATOSIS

This condition can result from sunlight exposure and occasionally occurs as a side effect of PUVA therapy when used as a treatment for other conditions and yet it responds to PUVA therapy. The therapeutic effect of PUVA therapy was confirmed by the controlled treatment of one patient who had an exacerbation of his condition after four treatments but finally cleared after 16 treatments. Bath PUVA therapy is also effective in clearing the disease.

URTICARIA

Urticaria is common and often refractory to treatment and mast cell function is altered by exposure to UV radiation, so it is curious that there are only a few studies of the effect of UV therapy on the various forms of urticaria. Most therapy centers do treat urticaria, particularly chronic idiopathic urticaria, and we need controlled trials to document the value of UV therapy.

Idiopathic

Chronic idiopathic urticaria responds to narrowband UVB phototherapy and to oral PUVA therapy producing clearance in about 50% of patients and improvement in another 20% in 20–40 treatments. Relapse is common and maintenance treatment is usually required.

Symptomatic Dermographism

A short course of UVB phototherapy relieved symptoms in the majority of patients with elimination of dermographism in many. In 50% of the patients, the remission lasted for at least 5 months. In contrast, a 4-week course of T.I.W. PUVA therapy produced improvement in less than half the patients, and there was no change in the dermographism; the course of treatment was probably insufficient.

Physical

Cold and aquagenic urticaria may respond to both PUVA and UVB phototherapy, but personal experience has indicated that PUVA therapy gives a faster and more complete response; maintenance requirements are variable.

Cholinergic

UVB phototherapy has been effective in a few reported cases.

Schnitzler Syndrome

This is a combination of bone pain, chronic urticaria, and recurrent fever. Narrowband UVB phototherapy and oral PUVA therapy can suppress the urticaria.

VASCULITIS

There is a report of two patients with idiopathic livedoid reticularis and livedoid vasculitis responding to brief courses of PUVA therapy with healing of ulcers and relief of symptoms; remissions lasted months. An explanation for this effect is not obvious but perhaps it ties in with the dramatic response of pigmented purpuras.

BIBLIOGRAPHY

Alopecia Areata

Claudy AL, Gagnaire D. Photochemotherapy for alopecia areata. Acta Dermatol Venereol (Stockh) 1979; 60:171–172.

Healy E, Rogers S. PUVA treatment for alopecia areata—does it work? A retrospective review of 102 cases. Br J Dermatol 1993; 129:42–44.

Larko O, Swanbeck G. PUVA treatment of alopecia totalis. Acta Dermatol Venereol (Stockh) 1983; 63:546–549.

Lassus A, Eskelinen A, Johansson E. Treatment of alopecia areata with three different PUVA modalities. Photodermatology 1984; 1:141–144.

Mitchell AJ, Douglass MC. Topical photochemotherapy for alopecia areata. J Am Acad Dermatol 1985; 12:644–649.

Taylor CR, Hawk JLM. PUVA treatment of alopecia areata partialis, totalis, and universalis: audit of 10 years' experience at St John's Institute of Dermatology. Br J Dermatol 1995; 133:914–918.

van der Schar WW, Sillevis Smitt JH. An evaluation of PUVA therapy for alopecia areata. Dermatologica 1984; 168:250–252.

Amyloidosis

Jin AGT, Por A, Wee LKS, Kai CKY, Leok GC. Comparative study of phototherapy (UVB) vs. photochemotherapy (PUVA) vs. topical steroids in the treatment of primary cutaneous lichen amyloidosis. Photodermatol Photoimmunol Photomed 2001; 17:42–43.

Darier's Disease

Sönnichsen VN, Brenke A, Diezel W. Dyskeratosis follicularis vegetans (Morbus Darier) therapie mit dem aromaitschen retinoid RO 10–9359 (Tigason®) in kombination mit systemischer photochemotherapie (ReUVA). Dermatol Monatsschr 1982; 168:520–522.

Dermatitis Herpetiformis

Kalimo K, Lammintausta K, Viander M. PUVA treatment of dermatitis herpetiformis. Photodermatology 1986; 3:54–55.

Eosinophillic Cellulitis

Diridl E, Hönigsmann H, Tanew A.Wells' syndrome responsive to PUVA therapy. Br J Dermatol 1997; 137:479–481.

Eosinophilic Fasciitis

Schiener R, Behrens-Williams SC, Gottlöber P, Pillekamp H, Peter RU, Kerscher M. Eosinophilic fasciitis treated with psoralen-ultraviolet A bath photochemotherapy. Br J Dermatol 2000; 142:804–807.

Eosinophilic Pustular Folliculitis

Buchness MR, Lim HW, Hatcher LA, Sanchez M, Soter NA. Eosinophilic pustular folliculitis in the acquired immunodeficiency syndrome. N Engl J Med 1988; 318:1183–1186.

Fearfield LA, Rowe A, Francis N, Bunker CB, Staughton RCD. Itchy folliculitis and human immunodeficiency virus infection: clinicopathological and immunological features, pathogenesis, and treatment. Br J Dermatol 1999; 141:3–11.

Porneuf M, Guillot B, Barneon G, Guilhou JJ. Eosinophilic pustular folliculitis responding to UVB therapy. J Am Acad Dermatol 1993; 29:259–260.

Rosenthal D, LeBoit PE, Klumpp L, Berger TG. Human immunodeficiency virus-associated eosinophilic folliculitis. Arch Dermatol 1991; 127:206–209.

Erythema Multiforme

Morison WL, Anhalt GJ. Therapy with oral psoralen plus UV-A for erythema multiforme. Arch Dermatol 1997; 133:1465–1466.

Erythrokeratoderma: Progressive and Symmetrical

Gheti P, DePadova MP, Bardazzi F. A case of erythrokeratodermia progressiva symmetrica: PUVA treatment. Case presentation, International Congress on Dermatology, Berlin, 1986.

Flegel's Disease

Cooper SM, George S. Flegel's disease treated with psoralen ultraviolet A. Br J Dermatol 2000; 142:340–342.

GVH Disease

Altman JS, Adler SS. Development of multiple cutaneous squamous cell carcinomas during PUVA treatment for chronic graft-versus-host disease. J Am Acad Dermatol 1994; 31:505–507.

Atkinson K, Weller P, Ryman W, Biggs J. PUVA therapy for drug-resistant graft-versus-host disease. Bone Marrow Transplant 1986; 1:227–236.

Aubin F, Brion A, Deconinck E, Plouvier E, Hervé P, Humbert Ph, Cahn JY. Phototherapy in the treatment of cutaneous graft-versus-host disease. Transplantation 1995; 59:151–155.

Elad S, Garfunkel AA, Enk CD, Galili D, Or R. Ultraviolet B irradiation. A new therapeutic concept for the management of oral manifestations of graft-versus-host disease. Lancet 1999; 88:444–450.

Hymes SR, Morison WL, Farmer ER, Walters LL, Tutschka PJ, Santos GW. Methoxsalen and ultraviolet: a radiation in treatment of chronic cutaneous graft-versus-host reaction. J Am Acad Dermatol 1985; 12:30–37.

Jampel RM, Farmer ER, Vogelsang GB, Wingard J, Santos GW, Morison WL. PUVA therapy for chronic cutaneous graft-versus-host disease. Arch Dermatol 1991; 127:1673–1678.

Kapoor N, Pellegrini AE, Copelan EA, Cunningham I, Avalos BR, Klein JL, Tutschka PJ. Psoralen plus ultraviolet A (PUVA) in the treatment of chronic graft versus host disease: preliminary experience in standard treatment resistant patients. Semin Hematol 1992; 29:108–112.

Leiter U, Kaskel P, Krähn G, Gottlöber P, Bunjes D, Peter RU, Kerscher M. Psoralen plus ultraviolet-A-bath photochemotherapy as an adjunct treatment modality in cutaneous chronic graft versus host disease. Photoderm Photoimmunol Photomed 2002; 18:183–190.

Vogelsang GB, Wolff D, Altomonte V, Farmer E, Morison WL, Corio R, Horn T. Treatment of chronic graft-versus-host disease with ultraviolet irradiation and psoralen (PUVA). Bone Marrow Transplant 1996; 17:1061–1067.

Volc-Platzer B, Hönigsmann H, Hinterberger W, Wolff K. Photochemotherapy improves chronic cutaneous graft-versus-host disease. J Am Acad Dermatol 1990; 23:220–228.

Wolff D, Anders V, Corio R, Horn T, Morison WL, Farmer E, Vogelsang GB. Oral PUVA and topical steroids for treatment of oral manifestations of chronic graft-vs-host disease. Photodermatol Photoimmunol Photomed 2004; 20:184–190.

Granuloma Annulare

Grundmann-Kollman M, Ochsendorf FR, Zollner TM, Tegeder I, Kaufmann R, Podda M. Cream psoralen plus ultraviolet A therapy for granuloma annulare. Br J Dermatol 2001; 144:996–999.

Hindson TC, Spiro JG, Cochrane H. PUVA therapy of diffuse granuloma annulare. Clin Exp Dermatol 1988; 13:26–27.

Kerker BJ, Huang CP, Morison WL. Photochemotherapy of generalized granuloma annulare. Arch Dermatol 1990; 126:359–361.

Granuloma Faciale

Hudson LD. Granuloma faciale: treatment with topical psoralen and UVA. J Am Acad Dermatol 1983; 8:559.

Histiocytosis X

Iwatsuki K, Tsugiki M, Yoshizawa N, Takigawa M, Yamada M, Shamoto M. The effect of phototherapies on cutaneous lesions of histiosytosis X in the elderly. Cancer 1986; 57:1931–1936.
Marchand C, Cambazard F, Kanitakis J, Thivolet J. Disseminated histiocytosis X: beneficial effect of phototherapy (PUVA) and topical mechlorethamine on cutaneous lesions. Case presentations. International Congress on Dermatology, Berlin, 1987.

Ichthyosis Linearis Circumflexa

Manabe M, Yoshiike T, Negi M. Successful therapy of ichthyosis linearis circumflexa with PUVA. J Am Acad Dermatol 1983; 8:905–906.
Nagata T. Netherton's syndrome which responded to photochemotherapy. Dermatologica 1980; 161:51–56.

Keratosis Lichenoides Chronica

Lang PG. Keratosis lichenoides chronica. Arch Dermatol 1981; 117: 105–108.

Lichen Planus

Gonzalez E, Momtaz T K, Freedman S. Bilateral comparison of generalized lichen planus treated with psoralens and ultraviolet A. J Am Acad Dermatol 1984; 10:958–961.
Helander I, Jansen CT, Meurman L. Long-term efficacy of PUVA treatment in lichen planus: comparison of oral and external methoxsalen regimens. Photodermatology 1987; 4:265–268.
Jansen CT, Lehtinen R, Happonen RP, Lehtnen A, Söderlund K. Mouth PUVA: new treatment for recalcitrant oral lichen planus. Photodermatology 1987; 4:165–166.
Kerscher M, Volkenandt M, Lehmann P, Plewig G, Röcken M. PUVA-bath photochemotherapy of lichen planus. Arch Dermatol 1995; 131:1210–1211.
Lundquist G, Forsgren H, Gajecki M, Emtestam L. Photochemotherapy of oral lichen planus. Oral Surg Oral Med Oral Pathol Oral Radiol Endod 1995; 79:554–558.

Naukkarinen A, Vaatainen N, Syrjanen KJ, Horsmanheimo M. Immuno-phenotyping of the dermal cells infiltrate in lichen planus treated with PUVA. Acta Derm Venereol (Stockh) 1985; 65:398–402.

Ortonne JP, Thivolet J, Sannwald C. Oral photochemotherapy in the treat-ment of lichen planus. Br J Dermatol 1978; 99:77–88.

Randle HW, Sander HM. Treatment of generalized lichen nitidus with PUVA. Int J Dermatol 1986; 25:330–331.

Lymphomatoid Papulosis

Volkenandt M, Kerscher M, Sander C, Meurer M, Röcken M. PUVA-bath photochemotherapy resulting in rapid clearance of lymphomatoid papulosis in a child. Arch Dermatol 1995; 131:1094.

Wantzin GL, Thomsen K. PUVA-treatment in lymphomatoid papulosis. Br J Dermatol 1982; 107:687–690.

Mastocytosis

Briffa DV, Eady RAJ, James MP, Gatti S, Bleehen SS. Photochemotherapy (PUVA) in the treatment of urticaria pigmentosa. Br J Dermatol 1983; 109:67–75.

Godt O, Proksch E, Streit V, Christophers E. Short-and long-term effective-ness of oral and bath PUVA therapy in urticaria pigmentosa and sys-temic mastocytosis. Dermatology 1997; 195:35–39.

Granerus G, Roupe G, Swanbeck G. Decreased urinary histamine metabo-lite after successful PUVA treatment of urticaria pigmentosa. J Invest Dermatol 1981; 76:1–3.

Kolde G, Frosch PJ, Czarnetzki BM. Response of cutaneous mast cells to PUVA in patients with urticaria pigmentosa: histomorphometric, ultrastructural, and biochemical investigations. J Invest Dermatol 1984; 83:175–178.

Mackey S, Pride HB, Tyler WB. Diffuse cutaneous mastocytosis. Arch Der-matol 1996; 132:1429–1430.

Ortonne JP, Forestier JY, Souteyrand P, Thivolet J. Mastocytes cutanés, histaminémie et photochimiothérapie orale. Ann Dermatol Venereol (Paris) 1980; 107:129–134.

Smith ML, Orton PW, Chu H, Weston WL. Photochemotherapy of domi-nant, diffuse, cutaneous mastocytosis. Pediatr Dermatol 1990; 7(4):251–255.

Necrobiosis

De Rie MA, Sommer A, Hoekzema R, Neumann HAM. Treatment of necrobiosis lipoidica with topical psoralen plus ultraviolet A. Br J Der-matol 2002; 147:743–747.

Ling TC, Thomson KF, Goulden V, Goodfield MJD. PUVA therapy in necrobiosis lipoidica diabeticorum. J Am Acad Dermatol 2002; 46:319–320.

McKenna DB, Cooper EJ, Tidman MJ. Topical psoralen plus ultraviolet. A treatment for necrobiosis lipoidica. Br J Dermatol 2000; 143:1333–1335.

Patel G. A prospective open study of topical psoralen-UV-A therapy for necrobiosis lipoidica. Arch Dermatol 2001; 137:1658–1661.

Papuloerythroderma

Bech-Thomsen N, Thomsen K. Ofuji's papuloerythroderma: a study of 17 cases. Clin Exp Dermatol 1998; 23:79–83.

Mutluer S, Yerebakan O, Alpsoy E, Ciftcioglu MA, Yilmaz E. Treatment of papuloerythroderma of Ofuji with re-PUVA: a case report and review of the therapy. J Eur Acad Dermatol Venereol 2004; 18:480–483.

Wakeel RA, Keefe M, Chapman RS. Papuloerythroderma. Arch Dermatol 1991; 127:96–98.

Perforating Dermatosis

Ohe S, Danno K, Sasaki H, Isei T, Okamoto H, Horio T. Treatment of acquired perforating dermatosis with narrowband ultraviolet B. J Am Acad Dermatol 2004; 50:892–894.

Pigmented Purpuric Dermatoses

Krizsa J, Hunyadi J, Dobozy A. PUVA treatment of pigmented purpuric lichenoid dermatitis (Gougerot-Blum). J Am Acad Dermatol 1992; 27:778–780.

Ling TC, Goulden V, Goodfield MJD. PUVA therapy in lichen aureus. J Am Acad Dermatol 2001; 45:145–146.

Wong WK, Ratnam KV. A report of two cases of pigmented purpuric dermatoses treated with PUVA therapy. Acta Derm Venereol (Stockh) 1991; 71:68–70.

Pityriasis Lichenoides

Boelen RE, Faber WR, Lambers JCCA, Cormane RH. Long-term follow-up of photochemotherapy in pityriasis lichenoides. Acta Derm Venereol (Stockh) 1982; 62:442–444.

Hofmann C, Weissman I, Plewig G. Pityriasis lichenoides chronica—eine neue Indikation zur PUVA-Therapie? Dermatologica 1979; 159:451–460.

LeVine MJ. Phototherapy of pityriasis lichenoides. Arch Dermatol 1983; 119:378–380.

Powell FC, Muller SA. Psoralens and ultraviolet A therapy of pityriasis lichenoides. J Am Acad Dermatol 1984; 10:59–64.

Thivolet J, Ortonne JP, Gianadda B, et al. Photochimiotherapie orale du parapsoriasis en gouttes. Dermatologica 1981; 163:12–18.

Pityriasis Rosea

Arndt KA, Paul BS, Stern RS, Parrish JA. Treatment of pityriasis rosea with UV radiation. Arch Dermatol 1983; 119:381–382.

Leenutaphong V, Jiamton S. UVB phototherapy for pityriasis rosea: a bilateral comparison study. J Am Acad Dermatol 1995; 33:996–999.

Valkova S, Trashlieva M,Christova P. UVB phototherapy for pityriasis rosea. J Eur Acad Dermatol Venereol 2004; 18:99–117.

Pruritus—Renal Failure

Blachley JD, Blankenship DM, Menter A, Parker TF, Knochel JP. Uremic pruritus: skin divalent ion content and response to ultraviolet phototherapy. Am J Kidney Dis 1985; 5:237–241.

Gilchrest BA, Rowe JW, Brown RS, Steinman T, Arndt KA. Ultraviolet phototherapy of uremic pruritus. Ann Intern Med 1979; 91:17–20.

Gilchrest BA, Rowe JW, Brown RS, Steinman TI, Arndt KA. Relief of uremic pruritus with ultraviolet phototherapy. N Engl J Med 1977; 297:136–138.

Saltzer EI. Relief for uremic pruritus: a therapeutic approach. Cutis 1975; 16:298–299.

Shultz BC, Roenigk HH. Uremic pruritus treated with ultraviolet light. J Am Med Assoc 1980; 243:1836–1837.

Stahle-Backdahl M. Uremic pruritus. Acta Derm Venereol (Suppl) (Stockh) 1989; 145:1–38.

Taylor R, Taylor AEM, Diffey BL, Hindson TC. A placebo-controlled trial of UV-A phototherapy for the treatment of uraemic pruritus. Nephron 1983; 33:14–16.

Pruritus—HIV Infection

Lim HW, Vallurapalli S, Meola T, Soter NA. UVB phototherapy is an effective treatment for pruritus in patients infected with HIV. J Am Acad Dermatol 1997; 37:414–417.

Pruritus—Polycythemia Vera

Baldo A, Sammarco E, Plaitano R, Martinelli V, Monfrecola G. Narrowband (TL-01) ultraviolet B phototherapy for pruritus in polycythaemia vera. Br J Dermatol 2002; 147:979–981.

Morison WL, Nesbitt JA. Oral psoralen photochemotherapy (PUVA) for pruritus associated with polycythemia vera and myelofibrosis. Am J Hematol 1993; 42:409–410.

Swerlick RA. Photochemotherapy treatment of pruritus associated with polycythemia vera. J Am Acad Dermatol 1985; 13:675–677.

Pruritus—Primary Biliary Cirrhosis

Cerio R, Murphy GM, Sladen GE, MacDonald DM. A combination of phototherapy and cholestyramine for the relief of pruritus in primary biliary cirrhosis. Br J Dermatol 1987; 116:265–267.

Hand MA, Levi AJ. Phototherapy for pruriritus in primary biliary cirrhosis. Lancet 1980; 2:530.

Perlstein SM. Phototherapy for primary biliary cirrhosis. Arch Dermatol 1981; 117:608.

Person JR. Ultraviolet A (UV-A) and cholestatic pruritus. Arch Dermatol 1981; 117:684.

Sclerosing Skin Diseases—Morphea

Grundmann-Kollmann M. Ochsendorf F, Zollner TM, Spieth K, Sachsenberg-Studer E, Kaufmann R, Podda M. PUVA—cream photochemotherapy for the treatment of localized scleroderma. J Am Acad Dermatol 2000; 43:675–678.

Kerscher M, Meurer M, Sander C, Volkenandt M, Lehmann P, Plewig G, Röcken M. PUVA bath photochemotherapy for localized sclero-derma. Arch Dermatol 1996; 132:1280–1282.

Morison WL. Psoralen UVA therapy for linear and generalized morphea. J Am Acad Dermatol 1997; 37:657–658.

Todd DJ, Askari A, Ektaish F. PUVA therapy for disabling pansclerotic morphoea of children. Br J Dermatol 1998; 138:201–202.

Sclerosing Skin Diseases—Systemic Sclerosis

El-Mofty M, Mostafa W, El-Darouty M, Bosseila M, Nada H, Yousef R, Esmat S, El-Lawindy M, Assaf M, El-Enani G. Different low doses of broad-band UVA in the treament of morphea and systemic sclero-sis. Photoderm Photoimmunol Photomed 2004; 20:148–156.

Hofer A, Soyer HP. Oral psoralen-UV-A for systemic scleroderma. Arch Dermatol 1999; 135:603–604.

Morita A, Sakakibara S, Sakakibara N, Yamauchi R, Tsuji T. Successful treatment of systemic sclerosis with topical PUVA. J Rheumatol 1995; 22:2361–2365.

Sclerosing Skin Diseases—Lichen Sclerosis et Atrophicus

Reichrath J, Reinhold J, Tilgen W. Treatment of genito-anal lesions in inflammatory skin diseases with PUVA cream photochemotherapy: an open pilot study in 12 patients. Dermatol 2002; 205(3):245–248.

Sclerosing Skin Diseases—Sclerodema

Grundmann-Kollman M, Ochsendorf F, Zollner TM, Spieth K, Kaufmann R, Podda M. Cream PUVA therapy for sclerodema adultorum. Br J Dermatol 2000; 142:1058–1059.

Hager CM, Sobhi HA, Hunzelmann N, Wickenhauser C, Scharenberg R, Krieg T, Scharffetter-Kochanek K. Bath-PUVA therapy in three patients with scleredema adultorum. J Am Acad Dermatol 1998; 38:240–242.

Sclerosing Skin Diseases—Scleromyxedema

Adachi Y, Iba S, Horio T. Successful treatment of lichen myxoedematosus with PUVA photochemotherapy. Photodermatol Photoimmunol Photomed 2000; 16:229–231.

Farr PM, Ive FA. PUVA treatment of scleromyxedema. Br J Dermatol 1984; 110:347–350.

Subacute Prurigo

Clark AR, C PA, Jorizzo JL, Fleischer AB. Papular dermatitis (subacute prurigo, "itchy red bump" disease): pilot study of phototherapy. J Am Acad Dermatol 1998; 38:929–933.

Sheretz EF, Jorizzo JL, White WL, Shar GG, C PA, Arrington J. Papular dermatitis in adults: subacute prurigo, American style? J Am Acad Dermatol 1991; 24:697–702.

Subcorneal Pustular Dermatosis

Cameron H, Dawe RS. Subcorneal pustular dermatosis (Sneddon-Wilkinson disease) treated with narrowband (TL-01) UVB phototherapy. Br J Dermatol 1997; 137:150–151.

Lubach D, Edmuller M, Rahm-Hoffman AL, Kombinierte retinoid und UV phototherapie bei pustulosis subcornealis (Sneddon-Wilkinson). Hautarzt 1980; 31:545–547.

Orton DI, George SA. Subcorneal pustular dermatosis responsive to narrowband (TL-01) UVB phototherapy. Br J Dermatol 1997; 137:149–150.

Park YK, Park HY, Bang DS, Cho CK. Subcorneal pustular dermatosis treated with phototherapy. Int J Dermatol 1986; 25:124–126.

Todd DJ, Bingham EA, Walsh M, Burrows D. Subcorneal pustular dermatosis and IgA paraproteinaemia: response to both etretinate and PUVA. Br J Dermatol 1991; 125:387–389.

Transient Acantholytic Dermatosis

Lüftl M, Degitz K, Plewig G, Röcken M. Bath psoralen-UV-A therapy for persistent Grover disease. Arch Dermatol 1999; 135:606–607.

Paul BS, Arndt KA. Response of transient acantholytic dermatosis to photochemotherapy. Arch Dermatol 1984; 120:121–122.

Urticaria

Berroeta L, Clark C, Ibbotson SH, Ferguson J, Dawe RS. Narrow-band (TL-01) ultraviolet B phototherapy for chronic urticaria. Clin Exp Dermatol 2004; 29:91–99.

Ciachini G, Colonna L, Bergamo F, Angelo C, Puddu P. Efficacy of psoralen-UV-A therapy in 3 cases of Schnitzler syndrome. Arch Dermatol 2001; 137:1536–1537.

Hannuksela M, Kokkonan EL. Ultraviolet light therapy in chronic urticaria. Acta Derm Venereol (Stockh) 1985; 65:449–450.

Johnsson M, Falk ES, Volden G. UVB treatment of facititious urticaria. Photodermatology 1987; 4:302–304.

Juhlin L, Malmros-Enander I. Familial polymorphous light eruption with aquagenic urticaria: successful treatment with PUVA. Photodermatology 1986; 3:346–349.

Logan RA, O'Brien TJ, Greaves MW. The effect of psoralen photochemotherapy (PUVA) on symptomatic dermographism. Clin Exp Dermatol 1989; 14:25–28.

Mideltart K, Moseng D, Kavli G, Stenvold SE, Volden G. A case of chronic urticaria and vitiligo, associated with thyroiditis, treated with PUVA. Dermatologica 1983; 167:39–41.

Vasculitis

Choi HJ, Hann SK. Livedo reticularis and livedoid vasculitis responding to PUVA therapy. J Am Acad Dermatol 1999; 40:204–207.

Special Situations

Some of the problems that arise during UV therapy for skin disease represent special situations, which the therapist must understand to arrive at the correct solution. Treating children is regarded by some as a problem in itself but this can easily be solved by an understanding of the potential pitfalls that arise.

20

Problem Cases

INTRODUCTION

The use of photons for therapy is very rewarding because almost all patients show a good response to treatment and thus you are interacting with patients who are pleased with the treatment. This situation is frequently magnified because many of the patients have been very displeased with their previous treatments. However, every patient does not have a problem-free course of treatment and it is necessary to have a good understanding of the potential problems to be able to intercede quickly as they arise. Participation in problem-solving clinics for phototherapy and photochemotherapy patients over many years, focused attention on several situations that frequently present as problems (Table 1). Together the problems discussed in this chapter account for about 95% of all patients discussed in that setting; therefore, although they have been mentioned elsewhere, they are worth special consideration.

THE NONRESPONDER

Clearance Failures

In the phototherapy and photochemotherapy of psoriasis vulgaris using regular protocols and no adjunctive therapy, some improvement should occur by the fifth or sixth treatment, and definite improvement should be seen by the 10th treatment. If this does not occur, the patient is classified as a slow

Table 1 Problem Cases

The Nonresponder
  Clearance failures
  Maintenance failures
Development of a new rash
Photosensitive psoriasis
Unusual erythemal responses
Alterations in pigmentation
HIV infection and psoriasis

responder. If no improvement is seen by treatment 20, or the patient has failed to achieve satisfactory clearing by treatment 30, the patient is classified as a nonresponder. Obviously, these statements are not to be applied rigidly; if a patient has been unresponsive to all other treatment and has no options, even a suggestion of a response may be a sufficient reason to continue. However, it is important to have a frame of reference so that consideration can be given to why the patient is not responding to treatment and steps can be taken to correct the situation. The reasons for a slow or failed response to treatment are as follows.

Missed Treatment

With both PUVA and UVB therapy, the most common reason for a failed response is missed treatments. Missing treatments permits the development of excessive pigmentation relative to the stage of therapy. The pigmentation of normal skin is only a guide because the fundamental problem is decreased transmission of radiation into the plaques of psoriasis, due to pigment that cannot be seen clinically. If the problem has not progressed too far, an accelerated schedule may permit the situation to be corrected. Frequently however, the only solution is to stop treatment until the pigment has cleared and then to start again as if with a new patient. The period of time off treatment depends on what treatment is being used: 4 weeks if on UVB phototherapy and 6–8 weeks if on PUVA therapy. Of course, the motivation and problems of the patient must be explored before deciding on either approach.

The Patient has a Tan

This is similar to the previous problem but the story is somewhat different. The patient may present in September with an exacerbation of psoriasis and may have spent the summer out boating, giving rise to a super tan. Alternatively, the patient may have been going to a tanning parlor for the past couple of months with minimal change in the extent of psoriasis but a major increase in pigmentation. Treatment should not be started in either case until the tan has cleared and if the disease is rapidly exacerbating, a combination protocol with acitretin or methotrexate should be considered. The problem of a tan can also arise during the clearance phase of treatment when a patient takes a vacation at the beach.

Low Cutaneous Methoxsalen Level

If there is a low level of methoxsalen in the skin, there will be a corresponding reduction of therapeutic effect. This situation must be suspected in the nonresponding patient who has little or no pigmentation of normal skin. There are several causes.

- Some patients do not take the medication and instead decide to try the effect of radiation without methoxsalen. This problem can be avoided by making it very clear during the initial consultation that neither the medication nor the radiation has any therapeutic effect alone, and by particularly emphasizing this point to patients who volunteer that they do not like taking drugs.
- The absorption of methoxsalen is low or delayed in up to 10% of patients. This can be confirmed by measuring the MPD, which will be abnormally high for the skin type of the patient, and then corrected by raising the dose of methoxsalen.
- Certain medications activate microsomal enzymes in the liver and enhance metabolism of methoxsalen. Carbamazepine, phenytoin, and phenobarbital are the common offenders and these drugs can prevent a therapeutic effect. Caution must be exercised if these medications are stopped because if the patient is having a high-exposure dose of UVA radiation, a major phototoxic effect can result from the sudden increase of active methoxsalen in the skin.

Unstable Psoriasis

Patients may present with very active inflammatory psoriasis or this may develop while on treatment. There are several causes.

- Long-term methotrexate treatment often leads to development of unstable psoriasis when the drug is withdrawn and this instability can persist for a year or more. There is no easy or guaranteed method for switching long-term methotrexate patients to UV therapy but the best approach is outlined in Table 2. The rebound of psoriasis that occurs in most patients coming off a long course of methotrexate usually begins 4 weeks after stopping the medication and reaches a peak at about 5 weeks, but an intensive level of UV treatment may be required for a longer period of time. The exacerbation of disease is most marked in areas that receive little exposure to radiation. The axillae, groin, and scalp are particularly

Table 2 Procedure for Changing from Long-Term Methotrexate Treatment to UV Therapy

---

Continue methotrexate, start PUVA plus UVB therapy
Clear disease and raise UV doses to a level suitable for the skin type
Stop methotrexate and continue clearance schedule at held doses of UV for 6–8
  weeks

---

affected, even if these areas were not involved prior to institution of methotrexate treatment. Some gradual improvement in these areas usually occurs with continued UV therapy, but complete remission is unusual. Another problem, which must be explained to the patient prior to changing treatments, is that UV therapy will not control associated arthritis or severe scalp involvement. If these two manifestations of psoriasis are of prime concern, it is probably preferable to continue with methotrexate therapy. An alternative approach is to use a low dose of methotrexate plus UV therapy, and this has the advantage of reducing the cumulative exposure to methotrexate and perhaps preventing, or certainly delaying, the appearance of liver toxicity. This treatment is often useful in patients with psoriatic arthritis since they usually only require a low dose of methotrexate to control joint symptoms.

- Lithium, antimalarials, and systemic corticosteroids all tend to make psoriasis unstable and often result in a failure to respond. Since these are likely to have been prescribed by another physician such as a psychiatrist or rheumatologist, direct questioning of the patient about other medications is required to uncover the problem. Combination therapy with, say, PUVA and methotrexate is usually required to suppress the psoriasis in these patients.

- Emotional stress in some patients can trigger instability in their psoriasis and, short of removing the cause of the stress, the only approach is to use aggressive treatment.

Koebner Phenomenon

In some patients with psoriasis, all areas clear quickly except for one or two persistent lesions. These patients should be asked whether the lesions are pruritic, because chronic scratching can produce a Koebner response and prevent clearance of the lesions. Often the patient will deny scratching the lesions, but a family member will sometimes volunteer that this does occur. The most common site for a persistence of plaques due to a Koebner phenomenon is on the front and sides of the legs. This is a very difficult problem, because it appears that neither UVB phototherapy nor PUVA therapy is very successful in clearing lesions in a patient who is having a Koebner response. One patient we treated for this problem was very insistent that she wanted her legs cleared of the disease for the summer months. Daily PUVA therapy plus daily anthralin treatment for 3 weeks was required to clear the disease at that site. Once the frequency of treatment was decreased, the lesions returned. Occlusive therapy of such lesions may provide some temporary improvement, but it is difficult to solve the problem completely.

Another cause of a Koebner phenomenon is occupational trauma, and this is usually seen on the dorsa of the hands in plumbers, carpenters, mechanics, and metal workers. Any patient with marked psoriasis at this site should be questioned about a likely cause since a hobby, such as wood carving, might be responsible. These patients require extra local exposure of the dorsa of the hands in a hand and foot machine to clear this site, and use of gloves to reduce the effect of trauma.

The Wandering Rash

Patients treated for localized disease, for example, on the palms and soles, occasionally develop lesions at distant, previously uninvolved sites during the course of treatment. This can occur with both eczema and psoriasis. For example, although the palms and soles may be responding well to PUVA therapy, the eruption appears on the forearms. Treatment for that site is followed by development of the eruption on the arms, and perhaps the face. Whole-body treatment is usually required at some point, and after control is achieved with this treatment, it is usually possible to revert to local treatment without recurrence at distant sites. The reason for this curious phenomenon is unknown, but it is almost as if the body has to express the disease somewhere.

Minimal Disease and Maximal Clearance

UV therapy should only be used in patients who have significant disease because treatment of minimal disease runs a high risk of the patient having the perception that the treatment is a failure. Most guidelines mention 10% or more of body-surface involvement as a minimal requirement. Obviously, the extent of disease is not the only factor that is important in determining whether a patient should be treated. Age, site of disease, and social disability are interrelated factors that must be considered. However, care must be exercised in patients with only minimal disease. Some patients with only 5% involvement will claim that their disease is such a disturbance to their lives that they must be treated. These patients can represent a problem because their expectation of the result of treatment tends to be higher than the physician anticipates or can achieve. Ninety percent improvement in a patient who started with 80% involvement of the body results in a very happy patient. Less than 100% improvement in a person with 5% involvement will usually result in an unhappy patient.

It is important to assess the expectations of the patient prior to the start of therapy and correct any misconceptions about the degree of clearance that will be achieved. Some patients not only expect 100% clearance but are very disappointed if that is not achieved. In most patients, even if 100% clearance is achieved, the maintenance requirements to retain a completely clear state are unacceptably high. For example, with PUVA therapy, one treatment every other week may keep a patient clear except for involvement of knees and elbows, whereas twice-a-week treatment may be necessary to keep these sites clear as well.

Misdiagnosis

In any patient not responding to a treatment, the possibility of an incorrect or missed diagnosis must be considered; fortunately, these are rare causes of failed UVB and PUVA therapy. Pityriasis rubra pilaris is probably the most common missed diagnosis accounting for psoriatic nonresponders, but this situation is rare. Psoriasiform SLE must also be considered. When treating diseases apart from psoriasis the range of possibilities broadens: scabies instead of atopic eczema, tinea and not eczema of the hands, secondary syphilis rather than pityriasis lichenoides et varioliformis acuta are a few to be considered.

Unknown Cause

When all these possibilities have been explored, there remains a group of patients who do not respond to treatment, and some other therapeutic approach must be tried. We have found that the PUVA-methotrexate protocol is very useful for nonresponders, and PUVA plus UVB therapy may also have value in these patients.

Maintenance Failures

The maximum frequency of maintenance treatment is usually considered to be Q.W. for PUVA therapy and B.I.W. for UVB phototherapy, and patients who require more frequent treatment to suppress their disease are maintenance failures. In the case of psoriasis, most patients have unstable disease and are difficult to clear. However, there are some patients who clear readily but flare up once they are put on a maintenance schedule.

The solution to the problem of maintenance failure is seldom easy and the options, from the most desirable to the least desirable, are as follows:

- If on UVB phototherapy, switch to PUVA therapy, or if on PUVA therapy, add UVB phototherapy.
- Use a combination of a low dose of methotrexate or acitretin plus PUVA therapy on a long-term basis.

- Change to another systemic agent.
- Accept the situation and use B.I.W. PUVA or T.I.W. phototherapy as maintenance treatment, but the situation should be re-evaluated frequently because such intense treatment is likely to be associated with an increased risk of skin cancer.

DEVELOPMENT OF A NEW RASH

Patients are on therapy for a rash and therefore are not entirely pleased when the treatment produces another rash. However, this does occur, and there are several types of eruptions that may be seen (Table 3).

Polymorphous Light Eruption

Considering the frequency of this disorder in a normal population, it is surprising that it only very occasionally develops during therapy. It may appear at any time, but most commonly develops during the clearance phase of treatment. If there is doubt about the correct diagnosis, it should be confirmed by histologic examination of a biopsy of the eruption plus immunofluorescent examination of skin. The best approach to polymorphous light eruption (PMLE) is to continue treatment to suppress the eruption and also clear the underlying disease being treated. If PMLE causes marked distress to the patient, a 10-day course of prednisone can be given to suppress the eruption while PUVA or UVB therapy is continued. Occasionally, PMLE will appear for the first time or reappear during maintenance therapy; consideration must then be given to changing wavebands of radiation for therapy.

Lupus Erythematosus

The development of lupus erythematosus (LE) on therapy is very rare, provided patients are screened for potential connective tissue disease at the initial evaluation, first on the basis of symptoms and if present, appropriate

Table 3 Rashes Complicating Treatment

Polymorphous light eruption
Lupus erythematosus
Transient acantholytic disease
Bullous pemphigoid
Guttate psoriasis
Seborrheic dermatitis
Porokeratosis
Actinic lichen planus
Chronic actinic dermatitis

investigation. However, this diagnosis must always be considered in the differential diagnosis of PMLE, in patients with photosensitive psoriasis, and in patients with unusual or unexplained erythemal responses. Fortunately, in the few patients who have developed subacute cutaneous LE under my care, there has been a complete remission once UV treatment has stopped.

Transient Acantholytic Disease

We have observed the development of transient acantholytic disease (TAD) in several patients on PUVA therapy, but the pathogenetic association is obscure. Usually, treatment can be continued which results in resolution of both TAD and the primary disease that is being treated. Occasionally, TAD will gradually worsen and rarely may become generalized, so that treatment has to be stopped.

Bullous Pemphigoid

A few patients have developed bullous pemphigoid while receiving UVB and PUVA therapy. This condition is a contraindication to further UV therapy. Bullae may develop on plaques of psoriasis during UVB phototherapy, but this is usually a manifestation of phototoxicity. If in doubt, immunofluorescent and histologic examination of a skin biopsy is necessary.

Guttate Psoriasis

The sudden appearance of a widespread papular eruption at any time during treatment should suggest the possibility of guttate psoriasis, presumably triggered by a respiratory infection or other stimulus. The best approach to this problem is to continue treatment.

Seborrheic Dermatitis of the Face

A complication of PUVA therapy is the appearance of a rash with the typical features of seborrheic dermatitis. The rash is usually confined to the central area of the face plus the eyebrows, but sometimes it involves the cheeks, and in this case it may resemble rosacea. Climatic and environmental factors appear to play a role in the etiology because it is most common at the change of seasons and can be very prevalent one year and almost nonexistent another year. The rash is exacerbated by PUVA therapy, and covering the face during treatment is helpful. Rapid clearance can be achieved by the combined use of a low-potency corticosteroid cream and a long-acting antifungal cream, and this treatment may have to be continued for some time to prevent a recurrence.

Porokeratosis

Disseminated superficial actinic porokeratosis can develop in a susceptible person on UV therapy and treatment should be stopped.

Actinic Lichen Planus

This is a very rare complication of UV therapy and also a reason for stopping therapy.

Chronic Actinic Dermatitis

This has been reported to occur as a complication of UV therapy and is probably coincidental, but its occurrence should raise the possibility of HIV infection since a CAD-type syndrome can be associated.

PHOTOSENSITIVE PSORIASIS

Some patients have psoriasis that exacerbates on exposure to sunlight or artificial UV radiation. A distinction must be made between photosensitive and photoirritable psoriasis. The condition of patients with very highly inflammatory disease, particularly in a pustular or erythrodermic phase, may be exacerbated by any trauma, and this is more correctly termed photoirritable psoriasis. The incidence of true photosensitive psoriasis is probably <1% of patients with psoriasis. The diagnosis should be suspected in any patient with involvement of the face with or without involvement of the hands and forearms.

Usually, the patient is aware of a direct exacerbation by sunlight or at least that the disease is worse in summer. Phototesting with UVA and UVB to determine an MED plus examination of the exposed sites 2–3 weeks later are helpful in diagnosis and management since a lowered MED to one waveband and production of lesions can suggest which treatment might be the safest.

The factors that play a role in the pathogenesis of photosensitive psoriasis are as follows.

Polymorphous Light Eruption

The development of this rash and subsequent Koebnerization is far and away the most common cause of photosensitive psoriasis. These patients can be treated with UV therapy, but it is absolutely essential to continue treatment when PMLE appears so as to suppress the eruption and prevent exacerbation of psoriasis. Topical corticosteroids and even systemic steroids are used if necessary for the comfort of the patient.

Skin Type I

These patients are more prone to develop erythema and again the mechanism of photosensitive psoriasis is probably via a Koebner response. The best approach to management is cautious treatment.

Vitiligo

Psoriasis and vitiligo are both common diseases, but in addition there is probably an association between them. As with skin type I patients, caution must be used when UV therapy is employed plus use of sunscreens on depigmented areas where this is feasible.

Lupus Erythematosus

The photosensitivity of LE may rarely be manifested as a psoriasiform eruption and this must be considered in all patients. A lupus package of serum tests is essential for all patients with photosensitive psoriasis, and further evaluation as indicated.

When these conditions have been excluded, there is still a small group of patients with photosensitive psoriasis that appears to be idiopathic in nature. These patients are best managed by an acitretin or methotrexate/PUVA schedule so that they are essentially desensitized by PUVA therapy while being suppressed by the systemic agent. Alternatively, a biologic agent may be the best approach for long-term management.

UNUSUAL ERYTHEMAL RESPONSES

Several normal erythemal responses are seen during treatment. During or immediately after exposure, erythema may appear, which lasts an hour or so. This response is probably immediate UV-induced erythema combined with heat erythema. The delayed phase of UVB-induced erythema is usually maximal at 8–12 hr and begins to regress after 18–24 hr. PUVA-induced erythema may peak at 48, 72, or as late as 96 hr after exposure.

Occasionally, patients give a history of other erythemal responses. Persistence of the immediate erythema may occur so that it lasts several hours. Every treatment, almost irrespective of dose, may cause erythema. Erythemal responses appearing several days after treatment are also a complaint in a few patients. The first consideration in patients with such problems must be latent SLE. A complete investigation for this disorder, including serum tests and immunofluorescent examination of a skin biopsy, is essential in these patients. Another possibility is that the patient is on a photosensitizing drug such as a thiazide. In addition, we have seen two patients who developed marked erythema after each PUVA treatment, with the only unusual feature of their presentations being concurrent medication with antimalarial drugs for arthritis. There is no obvious reason for this reaction, but both patients were forced to cease therapy. After all these diagnostic possibilities have been excluded, there remains a group of patients who have unusual erythemal responses of unknown cause. If the patient is significantly inconvenienced by the response, phototesting is necessary to determine if the response occurs with both PUVA and UVB radiation. The results will provide a guide to options for therapy.

ALTERATIONS IN PIGMENTATION

Treatment of certain diseases with UV therapy is associated with alterations in skin pigmentation at the site of the original lesions.

Depigmentation

Loss of pigmentation is most common in areas that were lichenified in patients with eczema and in patients with mycosis fungoides who had plaque-stage disease. Depigmentation can also develop occasionally in patients with acute or subacute eczema and lichen planus. The mechanism of the depigmentation is not known, but presumably the disease has caused a local disturbance of melanocyte function, and therefore it is a form of postinflammatory depigmentation.

The problem of depigmentation may not be immediately obvious because as lesions flatten, the skin just remains red, if that was the color of the lesions, or becomes pink to red. Complaints of pain and tenderness in the lesions may therefore be the first indications of the correct diagnosis. The problem then is to choose a dose of radiation that will control the disease and be tolerated by depigmented skin. When only a few lesions are depigmented, a broad-spectrum sunscreen can be applied to them before treatment to reduce the exposure dose, or zinc cream can be applied during treatment, so that only a portion of the total exposure dose is given to the affected sites. Widespread depigmentation usually requires shielding with clothing during part of the treatment.

Depigmentation has a variable prognosis. Some patients eventually develop normal pigmentation while treatment is continued, but only after 100 or more treatments. However, no significant recovery occurs in some patients despite several years of treatment and hundreds of exposures.

Hyperpigmentation

Temporary hyperpigmentation lasting a month or so is occasionally seen in any disease and all races treated with UV therapy. Persistent hyperpigmentation, often lasting years, is a feature of treatment of lichen planus in African–Americans or any person of skin types V and VI. Patients must be warned of this possibility before initiating treatment and this should be documented. Patients often regard the pigmentation as a scar and may sue the physician for leaving them scarred. One solution to the problem is to leave the patient on maintenance treatment every other week so that they maintain increased pigmentation of all skin and are at least one color. Depigmenting agents have no effect.

HIV INFECTION

UV therapy and HIV infection interact in a number of ways that can be important in treatment.

Effect of UV on HIV Infection

Exposure to UV radiation can activate HIV in in vitro culture systems and can stimulate replication of the virus in the skin of transgenic mice. The relevance of these findings to medical and environmental exposure to UV radiation in HIV-infected patients has been and remains very controversial. Several short-term studies have not found any adverse effect on viral load, CD-4 counts, or clinical progression from exposure to UVB phototherapy, or PUVA therapy. UV radiation is itself immunosuppressive, so there is the potential for inducing further suppression of the immune system in patients already compromised, but no evidence of this has been reported.

HIV Infection and Psoriasis

As immunosuppression becomes more marked in HIV-infected patients, previously stable psoriasis may exacerbate or psoriasis may appear for the first time and rapidly become very unstable. However, the incidence of psoriasis is not increased in HIV-infected persons and psoriasis in early stages of the infection can be present in mild and moderate forms. UV therapy can be useful in treating psoriasis in HIV-infected patients and if combination therapy is required, acitretin is the preferred agent. Methotrexate, which is immunosuppressive, is probably contraindicated.

UV Therapy of HIV-Associated Dermatoses

A number of dermatoses apparently triggered by HIV infection including eosinophilic folliculitis, pruritus, and a papular eruption, are responsive to UV therapy and have been treated with both UVB and PUVA therapy.

HIV Infection and Adverse Effects of UV

HIV-infected patients are immunosuppressed and other forms of immunosuppression are associated with an increased incidence of skin cancer. So far this does not appear to be a problem in patients treated with UV therapy, but as HIV-infected patients live longer lives due to successful treatment with protease inhibitors, this could emerge as a significant problem.

BIBLIOGRAPHY

The Nonresponder

Goldstein DP, Carter DM, Ljunggren B, et al. Minimal phototoxic doses and 8-MOP plasma levels in PUVA patients. J Invest Dermatol 1982; 78:429–433.

Wagner G, Hoffman C, Busch U, et al. 8-MOP plasma level in PUVA problem cases with psoriasis. Br J Dermatol 1979; 101:285–293.

Lupus Erythematosus

Bruze M, Krook G. Ljunggren B. Fatal connective tissue disease with antinuclear antibodies following PUVA therapy. Acta Dermatol Venereol (Stockh) 1983; 64:157–60.

Dowdy MJ, Nigra TP, Barth WF. Subacute cutaneous lupus erythematosus during PUVA therapy for psoriasis: case report and review of the literature. Arthritis Rheum 1989; 32:343–346.

Eyanson S, Greist MC, Brandt KD, Skinner B. Systemic lupus erythematosus. Arch Dermatol 1979; 115:54–56.

McFadden N. PUVA-induced lupus erythematosus in a patient with polymorphous light eruption. Photodermatology 1984; 1:148–150.

Millns JL, McDuffie FC, Muller SA, Jordan RE. Development of photosensitivity and an SLE-like syndrome in a patient with psoriasis. Arch Dermatol 1978; 114:1177–1181.

Bullous Pemphigoid

Abel EA, Bennet A. Bullous pemphigoid. Arch Dermatol 1979; 115:988–989.

George PM. Bullous pemphigoid possibly induced by psoralen plus ultraviolet A therapy. Photodermatol Photoimmunol Photomed 1995; 11:185–187.

Kuramoto N, Kishimoto S, Shibagaki R, Yasuno H. PUVA-induced lichen planus pemphigoides. Br J Dermatol 2000; 142:509–512.

Robinson JK, Baughman RD, Provost TT. Bullous pemphigoid induced by PUVA therapy. Br J Dermatol 1978; 99:709.

Thomsen K, Schmidt H. PUVA-induced bullous pemphigoid. Br J Dermatol 1976; 95:568–569.

Seborrheic Dermatitis

Tegner E. Seborrhoeic dermatitis of the face induced by PUVA treatment. Acta Dermatol Venereol (Stockh) 1983; 63:335–339.

Verhagen AR, Van Der Wiel AG, Wuite GG. Atypical psoriasis of the face and hands after PUVA treatment. Br J Dermatol 1984; 111:615–618.

Porokeratosis

Allen AL, Glaser DA. Disseminated superficial actinic porokeratosis associated with topical PUVA. J Am Acad Dermatol 2000; 43:720–722.

Hazen PG, Carney JF, Walker AE, Stewart JJ, Engstrom CW. Disseminated superficial actinic porokeratosis: appearance associated with photochemotherapy for psoriasis. J Am Acad Dermatol 1985; 12:1077–1078.

Actinic Lichen Planus

Wennersten G. Actinic lichenoid dermatitis induced by PUVA therapy in vitiligo patients. Photodermatology 1986; 3:247–248.

Chronic Actinic Dermatitis

Fujii N, Uetsu N, Hamakawa M, Futamura S, Okamoto H, Horio T. Chronic actinic dermatitis developed during phototherapy for psoriasis. Photodermatol Photoimmunol Photomed 2002; 18:157–159.

Photosensitive Psoriasis

Bielicky T, Kvicalova E. Photosensitive psoriasis. Dermatologica 1964; 129:339–348.

Doyle JA. Photosensitive psoriasis. Aust J Dermatol 1984; 25:54–58.

Ros AM, Eklund G, Odont D. Photosensitive psoriasis. J Am Acad Dermatol 1987; 17:752–758.

Ros AM, Wennersten G. Photosensitive psoriasis—clinical findings and phototest results. Photodermatology 1986; 3:317–326.

HIV Infection

Adams ML, Houpt KR, Cruz PD. Is phototherapy safe for HIV-infected individuals? Photochem Photobiol 1996; 64(2):234–237.

Beer JZ, Zmudzka BZ. UVB and PUVA therapies in HIV patients: are they safe? Photodermatol Photoimmunol Photomed 1997; 13:91–92.

Breuer-McHam J, Marshall G, Adu-Oppong A, Goller M, Mays S, Berger T, Lewis DE, Duvic M. Alterations in HIV expression in AIDS patients with psoriasis or pruritus treated with phototherapy. J Am Acad Dermatol 1999; 40:48–60.

Gelfand JM, Rudikoff D, Lebwohl M, Klotman ME. Effect of UV-B phototherapy of plasma HIV type 1 RNA viral level: a self-controlled prospective study. Arch Dermatol 1998; 134:940–945.

Horn TD, Morison WL, Farzadegan H, Zmudzka BZ, Beer JZ. Effects of psoralen plus UVA radiation (PUVA) on HIV-1 in human beings: a pilot study. J Am Acad Dermatol 1994; 31:735–740.

Meola T, Soter NA, Ostreicher R, Sanchez M, Moy JA. The safety of UVB phototherapy in patients with HIV infection. J Am Acad Dermatol 1993; 29:216–220.

Ranki A, Puska P, Mattinen S, Lagerstedt A, Krohn K. Effect of PUVA on immunologic and virologic findings in HIV-infected patients. J Am Acad Dermatol 1991; 24:404–410.

Stern RS, Mills DK, Krell K, Zmudzka Z, Beer JZ. HIV-positive patients differ from HIV-negative patients in indications for and type of UV therapy used. J Am Acad Dermatol 1998; 39:48–55.

21

Treatment of Children

INTRODUCTION

At times it appears that dermatologists and other physicians have overdone their anathema toward exposure to UV radiation and phototherapy in children is one of those situations. Often it is ignored as an option for treatment whereas in the same situation in an adult it would be the first option considered. Why? The answer is usually: children are so young, they have their whole life in front of them, and you should not expose them to a carcinogen. When the alternative is continued heavy exposure to corticosteroids or use of a potentially toxic systemic agent, UV therapy may be the best choice.

There are certain special considerations when exploring the option of UV therapy for children as well as a few tricks to make sure the treatment achieves a successful outcome and these will be considered here.

SELECTION OF PATIENTS

Who Are You Treating?

The first consideration when evaluating a child for UV therapy is to determine whether you are being asked to treat the disease in the child or the parent's concern about the disease in the child. Often you are going to treat both but also often a minor amount of disease which is not troubling the child will trigger parental concern that is out of proportion to the problem; in the latter situation do not treat.

Are the Logistics Favorable?

There are two aspects to this question. First, is the child's social calendar able to accommodate three trips to the office each week? Second, is someone available to bring the child to the office? If the answer to either question is no or maybe, delay treatment until there is a firm commitment to both.

Does the Child Want to be Treated?

If the answer to this question is no, do not bother to start treatment because it will almost certainly fail due to noncompliance. It is like piano lessons for a child who dislikes playing the piano, they will think up a dozen reasons for not coming in for treatment. The exception to this is when there are very compelling reasons to treat and then it is worth the effort to try and get cooperation.

Indications for Treatment

These are essentially the same as in adults with two exceptions:

- Children do not like applying topical agents so that UV therapy may be considered earlier than in adults.
- UV therapy may be considered as a steroid-sparing agent if there is evidence of growth retardation.

INTRODUCTION TO THE TREATMENT

Discussion with Parents

This should be more detailed than it is with most adults because you often have to deal with the "am I doing the right thing for my child" reaction. Short-term problems, the likely response to treatment and particularly the long-term risks of treatment must be discussed in detail.

Educating the Child

The child should be introduced to the treatment unit by the nurse or technician and be shown how it works and what they are expected to do. Likening the radiator to a "space machine" often captures their interest.

CHOICE OF TREATMENT

The initial dose of UV radiation is usually determined by skin type since it is not practical to do an MED test in a small child. The choice of treatment is mainly dictated by the disease being treated with a tendency to favor narrowband UVB phototherapy since it is simple to deliver and is perceived to have less long-term adverse effects.

Narrowband UVB Phototherapy

The main difference between use of this treatment in children and adults is that disease on the palms and soles is often responsive to the therapy in children due to thinner skin at these sites as compared to adults. It is not cost-effective to have a hand and foot area unit for the occasional child requiring treatment but instead the child can sit on a stool and point the palms and soles toward one bank of bulbs in a stand-up unit.

PUVA Therapy

PUVA therapy can be the treatment of choice in children in certain circumstances. When the disease is deep in the skin as in scleroderma, PUVA therapy is indicated since UVB radiation is less penetrating and it will not be effective. Pityriasis alba in patients with skin types III–VI is another situation where PUVA therapy is the treatment of choice due to its greater melanogenic effect. PUVA therapy should always be considered as an option even in very young children and its use will be determined by such factors as the effectiveness and toxicity of alternative treatments, the duration of therapy required, and the potential for adverse effects as suggested by characteristics of the patient such as skin type.

MECHANICS OF THE TREATMENT

Treating children with UV therapy does present some challenges and some of the common ones and their solutions deserve consideration.

Fear of Treatment

Children, and especially very young children, often find being left alone in a closed, brightly lit chamber a very scary experience. There are a couple of solutions for this. One, having the parent in the unit with the child for the first couple of treatments will often solve the problem. If UVB phototherapy is being used the parent will need protection by clothing and sunscreen while if PUVA therapy is used no special precautions are needed. The other is to keep the doors of the unit partly open with the parent sitting within view outside.

Ingestion of Psoralen

Young children may not be able to swallow capsules. The solution to this problem is to cut the capsule open and mix the solution inside with some peanut butter or jam and put it on some bread for the child to eat; the psoralen solution has a bad taste and hence it is necessary to disguise it. A strong caution: the parent must be instructed to wear gloves for protection from psoralen and to make sure the solution does not touch the child's lips since there is potential for marked phototoxicity.

Protection

When using PUVA therapy in children, eye protection is very important. The small goggles typically used during treatment provide adequate protection in the unit. For protection before and after treatment, inexpensive, wrap-around sunglasses labeled as being opaque to UV are available at many drug stores. During the treatment for all types of UV therapy, boys should wear boxer shorts and girls a pair of panties.

CONCLUSIONS

UV therapy is often the treatment of choice for many skin diseases in children because it offers rapid clearance and decreases the need for topical therapy, both big advantages for parents and children. If it is not suggested and offered by the physician, parents will often turn to use of a suntan parlor or sunlight and neither of these alternatives will provide a safe or effective treatment.

BIBLIOGRAPHY

Dohil M. UVB phototherapy in children. Pract Dermatol 2004; 4:28–32.
Holme SA, Anstey AV. Phototherapy and PUVA photochemotherapy in children. Photodermatol Photoimmunol Photomed 2004; 20:69–75.

New Therapies

Some new approaches to phototherapy have been introduced in the past decade and they are in a development phase. Lasers and other high-intensity light sources have become available to provide focused, local therapy of psoriasis and other skin diseases. UVA-1 phototherapy which was developed in Europe has been found useful for treating a limited number of skin diseases particularly atopic eczema. Finally, interest in treating acne with phototherapy has resurfaced after a thirty year hiatus of being ignored. These modalities are in a stage of evolution as their scientific and economic merits are being established. Studies are required comparing them to conventional therapies and in particular bilateral comparisons are essential to establish them as mainstream treatments.

22

Targeted Phototherapy with Lasers and Other High-Intensity Sources

INTRODUCTION

The concept of targeting phototherapy to the skin involved with disease is attractive for a number of reasons. First, it spares exposure of normal skin and thus reduces adverse effects. Second, in certain diseases such as psoriasis, involved skin has a higher tolerance to UV radiation as compared with uninvolved skin so that higher doses can be used. Third, since the discomfort of an erythema is limited to diseased skin, supraerythemogenic doses may be tolerated by the patient and such doses are known to clear disease faster than suberythemogenic doses. Application of this concept was limited until recently because reliable sources capable of delivering a large dose in a short period of time were not available. This changed with the development of the XeCL excimer laser, which generates 308 nm radiation. Several other high-intensity sources have now become available that are noncoherent and polychromatic.

Targeted phototherapy was initially used for the treatment of psoriasis but it is now being applied to treatment of a variety of other conditions; it can be assumed that all the diseases known to respond to UVB therapy will be responsive to this treatment. This leads to statement of a platitude which is easily forgotten in this high-technology world: in the absence of any thermal effects, there is no evidence that human skin can distinguish between a photon generated by a laser or other high-intensity source and a photon generated by a low-intensity source such as a fluorescent light bulb. The high-intensity sources discussed here do not generate thermal effects and the sole advantage of using them is that it permits delivery of a high dose in a short period of time. The rapid response reported with these high-intensity sources, as, for example, in repigmentation of vitiligo, is probably due to close attention to detail when treating small lesions so that erythema is maintained, rather than any inherent difference between these sources and a whole-body narrowband fluorescent radiator.

THE EXCIMER LASER

The Laser

The output of 308 nm radiation consists of a train of short, 20–40 nsec pulses at a pulse rate of up to 200 per second delivered through a liquid light guide (Xtrac laser, Photomedix, Carlsbad, CA). At this rate of delivery this is essentially a continuous wave laser. The beam cross-section is 3.24 cm (18 nm × 18 nm), the beam is fairly flat, the irradiance is 750 mW/cm^2, and the maximum output is over 4000 mJ per pulse. The laser can be used in a pulsed mode where a set dose is delivered for each pulse or a continuous mode where the dose delivered to skin depends on the operator moving the handpiece.

Psoriasis

This is a treatment for limited psoriasis of up to 2% body surface area since for larger areas the treatment becomes too long and tedious.

Treatment Schedules

Various protocols have been used and the dosimetry is still being investigated. The initial dose is based on a determination of the minimal erythemal dose (MED) of normal skin, a procedure, which takes only minutes to perform. Treatments are usually given twice weekly, starting with a multiple of the MED and increasing as tolerated. A medium-dose schedule of 2 × MED with 20% increments produces and maintains some erythema and clears most patients in about 10 treatments. A higher dose schedule (4 × MED) clears patients faster but produces painful erythema and blistering in some patients.

The laser is very useful in two areas that are usually difficult to treat with UV therapy. Scalp psoriasis responds very well. One study used a blower to separate the hair but after initially trying this technique we have found that manual separation of the hair is easier and more effective. A medium-dose schedule resulting in mild to moderate erythema on the scalp is usually tolerated without complaint. Inverse psoriasis is a second area that can respond very well to laser treatment since intertriginous areas are normally shielded during UV therapy.

Remissions

The duration of the remission following successful treatment with the excimer laser has been the subject of some debate. Since this is essentially narrowband UVB therapy, it would be anticipated that the average remission would be about 3 months and this has been our experience with some patients having a more rapid return of disease and some having much longer remissions.

Adverse Effects

Problems with the treatment are usually minor and limited to erythema. Painful erythema and blistering are uncommon except when using high-dose schedules but deserve caution since erosions can lead to a Koebner phenomenon. All patients who can pigment develop a tan, which some patients feel is unsightly, but it usually clears in 3–4 weeks.

Reimbursement and Costs

Procedure codes are now available (see Table 1) for this treatment and many insurance carriers, including Medicare, are providing reimbursement. In the United States the laser is mainly available on a pay-per-treatment basis, which has the advantages for the physician that there is minimal up-front cost and it is likely the laser will be regularly up-graded. The disadvantage of course is that you are always paying for the laser.

Other Diseases

There are few observations of a therapeutic effect of the excimer laser in other diseases.

Vitiligo

The treatment protocol is usually twice weekly treatments for 6 weeks to 6 months of therapy and doses used have resulted in mild erythema. Many patients have developed new perifollicular pigment but since the

Table 1 CPT Codes: 308 nm Excimer Laser for Psoriasis

CPT code
96920: Laser treatment for inflammatory skin disease (psoriasis); total area < 250 cm^2
96921: 250–500 cm^2
96922: Over 500 cm^2

repigmentation is rarely complete in the treated patients, it will probably be temporary. One study has shown that "UV unresponsive" areas such as the distal extremities are similarly unresponsive to laser treatment. Obviously, a bilateral comparison between laser treatment and conventional narrowband UVB therapy is required.

Hypopigmented Scars and Striae

Repigmentation of white striae and hypopigmented scars with improvement rates of 50–70% as compared to untreated control lesions judged by visual assessment has been observed after nine treatments. The pigmentation returned to baseline by 6 months so a course of maintenance treatment every month or two will be required to maintain a satisfactory cosmetic result.

Mycosis Fungoides

Four patients with patch stage (1A) mycosis fungoides had a clinical and histologic remission after a brief (4–11 treatments) course of therapy.

Alopecia Areata

Two patients had regrowth after about a dozen treatments.

Oral Lichen Planus

There are three reports of this condition responding in some patients after short courses of treatment.

Conclusions

Studies completed so far have clearly demonstrated that the excimer laser has a role in the treatment of localized psoriasis. Many questions remain about the treatment protocol, particularly concerning the frequency of treatment and dosage per treatment. This laser may also have a role in the treatment of other localized skin diseases. However, this requires a demonstration that a relatively expensive laser treatment is clearly superior to relatively inexpensive, and reimbursed, narrowband UVB therapy.

OTHER HIGH-INTENSITY SOURCES

Two devices capable of delivering high doses of UV radiation in very brief treatment times have received approval from the FDA. Both emit noncoherent and polychromatic radiation and are based on a mercury lamp. The systems run on 120 V power and both are readily portable.

The Devices

Dualight

This device emits either UVB (290–330 nm) or UVA (330–380 nm) with peaks at 335 and 365 nm) or a narrower spectrum around 311 nm. The radiation is delivered through a flexible light guide, the port is 3.61 cm^2 (19 nm × 19 nm square), and the irradiance for UVB is around 200 mW/cm^2. This device is available from Theralight Inc., Carlsbad, CA, or as the T500x from Daavlin, Bryan, OH.

B Clear or Relume

This device emits UVB (290–330 nm) radiation through a flexible light guide and the port is 2.56 cm^2 (16 nm × 16 nm square). The irradiance can be adjusted over a range of 50–800 mW/cm^2. This device is available from Lumenis Inc., Santa Clara, CA.

Indications

The two devices have been used to treat psoriasis, vitiligo, hypopigmented scars and striae, and eczema and although there is little published information there appears to be no reason to doubt their efficacy for targeted phototherapy.

Protocols

An MED can be determined easily with both devices and for psoriasis it is suggested they be used in supraerythemogenic mode starting at 2–6 × MED. The Dualight system can also be used in combination with Oxsoralen, either with a soak or with a lotion application, since it has a second waveband of UVA radiation.

Adverse Effects

These are the same as with the excimer laser: erythema, the potential for a Koebner phenomenon, and pigmentation.

Reimbursement and Cost

Reimbursement is through use of the phototherapy (96910) and PUVA therapy (96912) codes. This has an advantage over the laser codes of getting reimbursement for diseases other than psoriasis but the disadvantage that the amount of reimbursement is much lower. The devices can be bought outright. The devices can be used by any adequately trained person, whereas in a few states a laser can only be used by a physician.

Conclusions

There are no published studies comparing the excimer laser to these two nonlaser devices but, just by evaluating the specifications of the three systems, it would appear that efficacy should be fairly equal. A decision about which system to use is probably based on economics, portability, if that is a consideration, and whether a physician or another person is going to do the treatments.

BIBLIOGRAPHY

Psoriasis

Asawanonda P, Anderson RR, Chang Y, Taylor CR. 308 nm excimer laser for the treatment of psoriasis. Arch Dermatol 2000; 136:619–624.

Feldman SR, Mellen BG, Housman TS, Fitzpatrick RE, Geronemus RG, Friedman PM, Vasily DB, Morison WL. Efficacy of the 308 nm excimer laser for treatment of psoriasis: results of a multicenter study. J Am Acad Dermatol 2002; 46:900–906.

Gerber W, Arheilger B, Ha TA, Hermann J, Ockenfels HM. Ultraviolet B 308 nm excimer laser treatment of psoriasis: a new phototherapeutic approach. Br J Dermatol 2003; 149:1250–1258.

Mafong EA, Friedman PM, Kauvar ANB, Bernstein LJ, Alexiades-Armenakas M, Geronemus RG. Treatment of inverse psoriasis with the 308 nm excimer laser. Dermatol Surg 2002; 28:530–532.

Taneja A, Trehan M, Taylor CR. 308 nm excimer laser for the treatment of psoriasis. Arch Dermatol 2003; 139:759–764.

Taylor CR, Racette AL. A 308 nm excimer laser for the treatment of scalp psoriasis. Lasers Surg Med 2004; 34:136–140.

Tournas JA, Lowe NJ, Yamauchi PS. Laser and novel light source treatments for psoriasis. Lasers Surg Med 2004; 35:165–173.

Trehan M, Taylor CR. Medium-dose 308 nm excimer laser for the treatment of psoriasis. J Am Acad Dermatol 2002; 47:701–708.

Vitiligo

Baltás E. Treatment of vitiligo with the 308 nm xenon chloride excimer laser. Arch Dermatol 2002; 138:1619–1620.

Esposito M, Soda R, Costanzo A, Chimenti S. Treatment of vitiligo with the 308 nm excimer laser. Clin Exp Dermatol 2004; 29:133–137.

Grimes PE. Advances in the treatment of vitiligo: targeted phototherapy. Cosmet Dermatol 2003; 16:18–22.

Ostovari N, Passeron T, Zakaria W, Fontas E, Larouy JC, Blot JF, Lacour JPh, Ortonne JP. Treatment of vitiligo by 308 nm excimer laser: an evaluation of variables affecting treatment response. Lasers Surg Med 2004; 35:152–156.

Spencer JM, Nossa R, Ajmeri J. Treatment of vitiligo with the 308 nm excimer laser: a pilot study. J Am Acad Dermatol 2002; 46:727–731.

Other Diseases

Alexiades-Armenakas MR, Bernstein LJ, Friedman PM, Geronemus RG. The safety and efficacy of the 308 nm excimer laser for pigment correction of hypopigmented scars and striae alba. Arch Dermatol 2004; 140:955–960.

Friedman PM, Geronemus RG. Use of the 308 nm excimer laser for postresurfacing leukoderma. Arch Dermatol 2001; 137:824–825.

Goldberg DJ, Sarradet D, Hussain M. 308 nm excimer laser treatment of mature hypopigmented striae. Dermatol Surg 2003; 29:596–599.

Gundogan C, Greve B, Raulin C. Treatment of alopecia areata with the 308 nm xenon chloride excimer laser: case report of two successful treatments with the excimer laser. Lasers Surg Med 2004; 34:86–90.

Köllner K, Wimmershoff M, Landthaler M, Hohenleutner U. Treatment of oral lichen planus with the 308 nm UVB excimer laser—early preliminary results in eight patients. Lasers Surg Med 2003; 33:158–160.

Mori M, Campolmi P, Mavilia L, Rossi R, Cappugi P, Pimpinelli N. Monochromatic excimer light (308 nm) in patch-stage IA mycosis fungoides. J Am Acad Dermatol 2004; 50:943–945.

Passeron T, Zakaria W, Ostovari N, Mantoux F, Lacour JPH, Ortonne JP. Treatment of erosive oral lichen planus by the 308 nm excimer laser. Lasers Surg Med 2004; 34:205.

Trehan M, Taylor CR. Low-dose excimer 308-nm laser for the treatment of oral lichen planus. Arch Dermatol 2004; 140:415–420.

23

UVA-1 Phototherapy

INTRODUCTION

There has been marked interest in the past few years in the therapeutic potential of UVA-1 (340–400 nm) radiation with lots of reports of benefit in a variety of diseases. Most of the reports have been from Europe where a few centers have metal halide devices capable of generating high irradiances, which are necessary to keep treatment times at a reasonable level. Controlled studies have been conducted in a few diseases such as atopic eczema, scleroderma, and lupus erythematosus but in other conditions there are mainly case reports or small series.

UVA-1 phototherapy is divided into low-dose (10–30 J/cm^2 per exposure), medium-dose, (50–60 J/cm^2 per exposure), and high-dose (130 J/cm^2). There is evidence in some conditions that efficacy is dependent on dose but more study is required to establish this as fact. In addition, more studies are required to establish superiority of UVA-1 phototherapy over more readily available treatments such as PUVA therapy and UVB phototherapy.

UVA-1 phototherapy has not attracted a lot of interest in the USA for several reasons. First, the treatment units for whole-body exposure are large and take a lot of treatment space. Second, the units are expensive, costing more than four times the cost of a stand-up UV radiator. Third, reimbursement is the same as for any other form of phototherapy. Finally, no clear advantage of the treatment has been demonstrated in any disease so it appears unlikely that a constituency will emerge to support a new reimbursement code in the near future.

INDICATIONS

Diseases reported to respond to UVA-1 phototherapy are listed in Table 1.

Atopic Eczema

High-dose ($130\,\mathrm{J/cm^2}$) and medium-dose ($50\,\mathrm{J/cm^2}$) UVA-1 phototherapy given daily, five times a week for 3 weeks are effective in acute, severe atopic dermatitis and in this situation are superior to UVA-B phototherapy, moderate-potency corticosteroids, or low-dose ($20\,\mathrm{J/cm^2}$) UVA-1 phototherapy. The duration of remission from this treatment is brief with most patients relapsing to pretreatment condition in 1–3 months. It has been suggested that patients should be switched to narrowband UVB phototherapy after

Table 1 Response of Various Dermatoses to UVA-1 Phototherapy

	Controlled Trial	Open Trial	Anecdote
Atopic eczema	+++		
Localized scleroderma	+++		
Systemic lupus erythematosus	++		
PMLE prophylaxis	++		
Mycosis fungoides		+++	
Urticaria pigmentosa		+++	
Scleredema		+++	
Systemic sclerosis		++	
Hypereosinophilic syndrome		++	
Graft-versus-host disease		++	
Vesicular hand eczema		++	
Granuloma annulare		++	
Lichen sclerosis		++	
Pityriasis lichenoides			++
Keloids			+
Sarcoid			+
Vitiligo			−
Psoriasis			−
Acne			−

Note: +++, complete clearance; ++, partial clearance; +, minimal response; −, no response.

treatment with UVA-1 phototherapy to prolong the remission but this approach does not appear to have been studied in a trial.

Scleroderma

Localized scleroderma (widespread morphea, pansclerotic morphea, and linear morphea) has been successfully treated with low-, medium- and high-dose UVA-1 phototherapy with some evidence that a high-dose schedule of 30 exposures to $130 \, \text{J/cm}^2$ over 10 weeks is superior to a low-dose schedule of $20 \, \text{J/cm}^2$. The cutaneous changes in systemic scleroderma, including acrosclerosis, are also improved by treatment.

Systemic Lupus Erythematosis

Low-dose ($6 \, \text{J/cm}^2$) UVA-1 phototherapy has been found in two randomized trials to be effective in reducing disease activity and antibody levels without significant side effects. Photosensitivity was not a problem and indeed this has been found to improve in patients with the subacute form of LE.

Mycosis Fungoides

Several case reports and one series of 13 patients have found very encouraging results from UVA-1 phototherapy even in patients with tumors. Persistence of lesions in sanctuary sites indicates the effect of treatment is local and provides some element of "control" for these observations.

ADVERSE EFFECTS

Erythema

The doses of UVA-1 used can be very high and will exceed the erythema threshold in some patients. It is therefore essential to do an MED before commencing treatment and the initial dose will be guided by the results.

Pigmentation

UVA-1 therapy induces a marked tanning response and when treating morphea, this can be accentuated in resolving lesions.

Skin Cancer

UVA-1 radiation does produce DNA damage and has produced tumors in mice. These findings raise the question of its carcinogenic potential in humans, particularly because there is some evidence that longer wavelengths may favor development of melanoma skin cancer.

MECHANISM OF ACTION

The mechanism by which UVA-1 radiation produces a therapeutic effect probably varies in different diseases. In atopic eczema and mycosis fungoides, apoptosis of skin-infiltrating T helper cells through an oxygen dependent pathway is a likely mechanism. Reduction in the number of Langerhans cells and mast cells could also be important in atopic eczema and mast cell depletion is the likely mechanism in urticaria pigmentosa. In scleroderma and keloids, increased expression of collagenase is a possible mechanism.

EQUIPMENT

Two systems are available.

High-Output System

Several systems capable of delivering high-dose and medium-dose UVA-1 phototherapy are available in Europe but only one lighting company (Daavlin, Bryan, OH) sells this equipment in the USA. The systems use a metal halide lamp with a short-wavelength cutoff filter to remove wavelengths below 340 nm and a long-wavelength filter to remove most of the visible light and infrared radiation. An area unit containing one lamp is suitable for treating a local area of about 1 ft^2. The whole-body unit contains 12 lamps and is a lie-down unit. There are several considerations with the whole-body unit.

Size

The lie-down unit is 92 in long and 54 in wide, so its imprint is equivalent to a couple of stand-up units.

Heat Load

A considerable heat load is generated by this system and this must be ducted to the exterior and combined with the use of additional air-conditioning for patient comfort.

Treatment Times

The lamps are only on one side, above the patient, so treatment time is doubled when using a whole-body treatment. Thus, for a dose of 130 J/cm^2 the treatment time will be 48–60 min at an irradiance of 70–90 mW/cm^2.

Low-Output System

For delivery of low-dose UVA-1 therapy any stand-up UV radiator can be easily converted by substituting TL/ 10 R lamps (Philips Lighting,

Eindhoven, The Netherlands) and inserting a UVASUN or similar plastic filter between the lamps and the patient. This will provide an irradiance of about $20\,mW/cm^2$ in the UVA-1 waveband so that a $20\,J/cm^2$ treatment will take about 16 min.

CONCLUSIONS

UVA-1 phototherapy is clearly in a development phase in its evolution as a potential treatment and much more work needs to be done to establish its value. Further investigation of the dose-dependency issue is required. High-, medium- and low-dose schedules have been compared but the efficacy of a low-dose schedule given daily over a longer period, resulting in the same high total dose, has not been addressed. More bilateral comparisons with narrowband UVB phototherapy and PUVA therapy are also required to place this new treatment in the context of established and readily available treatments. Finally, if medium- and high-dose schedules are essential for successful therapy, economic considerations are likely to impede its widespread use in the United States.

BIBLIOGRAPHY

Reviews

Dawe RS. Ultraviolet A1 phototherapy. Br J Dermatol 2003; 148:626–637.

Atopic Eczema

Abeck D, Schmidt T, Fesq H, Strom K, Mempel M, Brockow K, Ring J. Long-term efficacy of medium-dose UVA1 phototherapy in atopic dermatitis. J Am Acad Dermatol 2000; 42:254–257.

Kowalzick L, Kleinheinz A, Weichenthal M, Neuber K, Köhler I, Grosch J, Lungwitz G, Seegeberg C, Ring J. Low dose versus medium dose UV-A1 treatment in severe atopic eczema. Acta Derm Venereol (Stockh) 1995; 75:43–45.

Krutmann J. Phototherapy for atopic dermatitis. Dermatol Ther 1996; 1:24–31.

Krutmann J, Diepgen TL, Luger TA, Grabbe S, Meffert H, Sönnichsen N, Czech W, Kapp A, Stege H, Grewe M, Schöpf E. High-dose UVA1 therapy for atopic dermatitis: results of a multicenter trial. J Am Acad Dermatol 1998; 38:589–593.

Krutmann J, Czech W, Diepgen T, Niedner R, Kapp A, Schöpf E. High-dose UVA1 therapy in the treatment of patients with atopic dermatitis. J Am Acad Dermatol 1992; 26:225–230.

Von Kobyletzki G, Pieck C, Hoffmann K, Freitag M, Altmeyer P. Medium-dose UVA1 cold-light phototherapy in the treatment of severe atopic dermatitis. J Am Acad Dermatol 1999; 41:931–937.

Tzaneve S, Seeber A, Schwaiger M, Hönigsmann H, Tanew D. Comparative efficacy of high-dose versus medium-dose UVA1 phototherapy for patients with severe, generalized atopic dermatitis. J Am Acad Dermatol 2001; 45:503–507.

Scleroderma

Camacho NR, Sanchez JE, Martin RF, González JR, Sánchez JL. Medium-dose UVA1 phototherapy in localized scleroderma and its effect in CD34-positive dendritic cells. J Am Acad Dermatol 2001; 45:697–699.

Gruss CJ, von Kobyletzki G, Behrens-Williams SC, Lininger J, Reuther T, Kerscher M, Altmeyer P. Effects of low dose ultraviolet A-1 phototherapy on morphea. Photodermatol Photoimmunol Photomed 2001; 17:149–155.

Kerscher M, Volkenandt M, Gruss C, Reuther T, von Kobyletzki G, Freitag M, Dirschka T, Altmeyer P. Low-dose UVA$_1$ phototherapy for treatment of localized scleroderma. J Am Acad Dermatol 1998; 38:21–26.

Von Kobyletzki G. Acrosclerosis in patients with systemic sclerosis responds to low-dose UV-A1 phototherapy. Arch Dermatol 2000; 136:275–276.

Kreuter A, Breuchmann F, Uhle A, Brockmeyer N, von Kobyletzki G, Freitag M, Stuecker M, Hoffman K, Gambichler T, Altmeyer P. Low-dose UVA1 phototherapy in systemic sclerosis: effects on acrosclerosis. J Am Acad Dermatol 2004; 50:740–747.

Morita A, Kobayashi K, Isomura I, Tsuji T, Krutmann J. Ultraviolet A1 (340–400 nm) phototherapy for scleroderma in systemic sclerosis. J Am Acad Dermatol 2000; 43:670–674.

Steger JW. UVA therapy for scleroderma. J Am Acad Dermatol 1999; 40:787.

Stege H, Berneburg M, Humke S, Klammer M, Grewe M, Grether-Beck S, Boedeker R, Diepgen T, Dierks K, Goerz G, Ruzicka T, Krutmann J. High-dose UVA$_1$ radiation therapy for localized scleroderma. J Am Acad Dermatol 1997; 36:938–944.

Systemic Lupus Erythematosus

McGrath H. Ultraviolet-A1 irradiation decreases clinical disease activity and autoantibodies in patients with systemic lupus erythematosus. Clin Exp Rheumatol 1994; 12:129–135.

McGrath H. UV-A1 light decreases disease activity and eliminates antibodies in patients with systemic lupus erythematosus. In: Urbach F, ed. Biological Responses to UVA Radiation. Overland Park, KS: Valdenmar Publ. Co., 1992:257–260.

McGrath H, Martinez-Osuna P, Akdamar F. Ultraviolet-A1 (340–400°nm) irradiation therapy in systemic lupus erythematosus. Lupus 1996; 5(4):269–274.

Molina JF, McGrath H. Longterm ultraviolet-A1 irradiation therapy in systemic lupus erythematosus. J Rheumatol 1997; 24:1072–1074.

Sönnichsen N, Meffert H, Kunzelmann V, Audring H. UV-A-1 therapie bei subakut-kutanem lupus erythematodes. Hautarzt 1993; 44:723–725.

Mycosis Fungoides

Plettenberg H, Stege H, Megahed M, Ruzicka T, Hosokawa Y, Tsuji T, Morita A, Krutmann J. Ultraviolet A1 (340–400°nm) phototherapy for cutaneous T-cell lymphoma. J Am Acad Dermatol 1999; 41:47–50.

Von Kobyletzki G, Heine O, Stephan H, Pieck C, Stücker M, Hoffmann K, Altmeyer P, Mannherz HG. UVA1 irradiation induces deoxyribonuclease dependent apoptosis in cutaneous T-cell lymphoma in vivo. Photodermatol Photoimmunol Photomed 2000; 16:271–277.

Zane C, Leali C, Airò P, De Panfilis G, Calzavara Pinton P. "High-dose" UVA1 therapy of widespread plaque-type, nodular, and erythrodermic mycosis fungoides. J Am Acad Dermatol 2001; 44:629–633.

Other Diseases

Asawanonda P, Khoo LSW, Fitzpatrick TB, Taylor CR. UV-A1 for keloid. Arch Dermatol 1999; 135:348–349.

Grundmann-Kollmann M, Behrens S, Gruss C, Gottlöber P, Peter RU, Kerscher M. Chronic sclerodermic graft-versus-host disease refractory to immunosuppressive treatment responds to UVA$_1$ phototherapy. J Am Acad Dermatol 2000; 42:134–136.

Janinga JJ, Ward DH, Lim HW. UVA-1 as a treatment for scleroderma. Photodermatol Photoimmunol Photomed 2004; 20:210–211.

Kreuter A, Gambichler T, Avermaete A, Happe M, Bacharach-Buhles M, Hoffman K, Jansen T, Altmeyer P, von Kobyletzki G. Low-dose ultraviolet A1 phototherapy for extragenital lichen sclerosus: results of a preliminary study. J Am Acad Dermatol 2002; 46:251–255.

Mahnke N, Medve-Koenigs K, Berneburg M, Ruzicka T, Neumann NJ. Cutaneous sarcoidosis treated with medium-dose UVA1. J Am Acad Dermatol 2004; 50:978–979.

Meewes C, Henrich A, Krieg T, Hunzelmann N. Treatment of reticular erythematosus mucinosis with UV-A1 radiation. Arch Dermatol 2004; 140:660–662.

Muchenberger S, Schöpf E, Simon JC. Phototherapy with UV-A-1 for generalized granuloma annulare. Arch Dermatol 1997; 133:1605.

Petering H, Breuer C, Herbst R, Kapp A, Werfel T. Comparison of localized high-dose UVA1 irradiation versus topical cream psoralen-UVA for treatment of chronic vesicular dyshidrotic eczema. J Am Acad Dermatol 2004; 50:68–72.

Plötz SG, Abeck D, Seitzer U, Hein R, Ring J. UVA1 for hypereosinophilic syndrome. Acta Derm Venereol 2000; 80:221.

Ständer H, Schiller M, Schwarz T. UVA1 therapy for sclerodermic graft-versus-host disease of the skin. J Am Acad Dermatol 2002; 46:799–800.

Stege H, Schöpf E, Ruzicka T, Krutmann J. High-dose UVA1 for urticaria pigmentosa. Lancet 1996; 347:64.

Ziemer M, Thiele JJ, Grubn B, Elsner P. Chronic cutaneous graft-versus-host disease in two children responds to UVA1 therapy: improvement of skin lesions, joint mobility, and quality of life. J Am Acad Dermatol 2004; 51:318–319.

24

Phototherapy of Acne Vulgaris

INTRODUCTION

Acne vulgaris is a disease of sebaceous glands characterized by comedones, papules, pustules, and cystic lesions and has a complex pathophysiology including

- Hyperkeratinization of the neck of the hair follicle and of the sebaceous duct resulting in obstruction
- Increased production of sebum
- Increased free fatty acid content of sebum due to bacterial activity, predominantly by propionibacterium acnes
- Often rupture of the follicle and release of sebum and keratin into the dermis
- Inflammation
- An influence by hormonal and climatic factors and emotional stress.

Interest in using photons to interrupt or prevent this cascade of events is usually attributed to the observation that acne often improves during summer and a belief, by physicians and patients, that sunlight helps to clear acne; there are no studies to support this belief. Sunlight is a very complex environment involving exposure to multiple wavebands of radiation, often in a relaxed or hormone-stimulating setting and it can induce tanning, which will camouflage acne lesions. A further complication is that about 20% of patients with acne are made worse by exposure to sunlight.

Studies have evaluated the efficacy of UVB, UVA, UVA plus UVB, topical PUVA, and oral PUVA using counts of lesions as the end point and no significant benefit was seen. Patients who tanned were usually pleased with treatment, which suggests the camouflage effect can be important. Recently, there has been a resurgence of interest in using phototherapy and lasers to treat acne so that almost every throwaway publication has news about a new light source being used successfully. Unfortunately, there have been few bilateral comparison studies of these treatments and this should be the gold standard for determining efficacy.

TREATMENTS

Three principal targets have been used for treatment: the sebaceous gland, the vascular component of inflammation, and propionibacterium acnes. It is very likely that the mechanism of action of all the proposed treatments is much more complex than is presently understood.

The Sebaceous Glands

Removal of all sebaceous glands will eliminate acne but the long-term consequences of doing this are unknown and therefore a more conservative approach of shrinking the size of glands and targeting involved glands has been adopted.

Diode Laser (1450 nm)

A diode laser (Smoothbeam®, Candela Corporation, Wayland, MD) with an emission of 1450 nm and a cooling device to protect the epidermis produced a highly significant reduction in lesion count after one treatment and a greater reduction after four treatments. This effect was sustained for 24 weeks after the last treatment. There were no significant adverse effects. The chromophore is water and the long wavelength of this laser allows penetration to the level of the sebaceous glands.

Exogenous Photodynamic Therapy

Topical application of aminolevulinic acid and subsequent exposure to broadband (550–700 nm) visible light has been found effective in improving acne to a considerable degree. The sensitizer does accumulate in the glands and is converted to protoporphyrin. Shrinkage of glands and decreased sebum production was found and benefit lasted beyond 6 months. However, this treatment is associated with pain during the procedure, crusting and discomfort for 10–20 days, and pigmentation for months. There are anecdotal reports of the use of other light sources and lasers with less morbidity, but efficacy has not been documented in controlled studies.

The Inflammatory Component

A pulsed-dye laser has been used to presumably eliminate blood vessels in lesions with anecdotal reports of good sustained results. However, a randomized split-face study found the treatment to be ineffective.

Propionibacterium Acnes

This bacterium produces porphyrins, mainly coproporphyrin III, with an absorption spectrum around 415 nm, raising the possibility of inducing endogenous photodynamic therapy with this photosensitizer. Two light sources are approved by the FDA for treating acne using this approach.

Clearlight

This is a narrowband (407–420 nm) metal halide lamp (Lumenis, Santa Clara, CA), which in uncontrolled studies produced a 60–70% reduction of inflammatory lesions after 10 treatments. In an unpublished split-face study in 66 patients, 32% improved only on the treated side after eight treatments.

Omnilux-Blue

This is an LED light source emitting at 415 nm (Alderm, Irvine, CA), which in unpublished studies produced about 60% reduction of inflammatory lesions after eight treatments; there were no controls.

CONCLUSIONS

There is new interest in the use of photons to treat acne and that is welcome news. However, there are several reservations to keep in mind. More work is needed on the mechanisms by which these treatments work so the treatments can be optimized. Each treatment requires confirmation of efficacy in bilateral-comparison randomized trials because acne is a notoriously variable condition with patients improving and deteriorating in the absence of any treatment. A phototherapy treatment will be preferable to a laser treatment from an economic standpoint since it would likely be at a lower cost.

BIBLIOGRAPHY

Cunliffe WJ, Goulden V. Phototherapy and acne vulgaris. Br J Dermatol 2000; 142:855–856.

Hirsch RJ, Shalita AR. Lasers, light, and acne. Cutis 2003; 71:353–354.

Hongcharu W, Taylor CR, Chang Y, Aghassi D, Suthamjariya K, Anderson RR. Topical ALA-photodynamic therapy for the treatment of acne vulgaris. J Invest Dermatol 2000; 115:183–192.

Itoh Y, Ninomiya Y, Tajima S, Ishibashi A. Photodynamic therapy of acne
    vulgaris with topical 8-aminolaevulinic acid and incoherent light in
    Japanese patients. Br J Dermatol 2001; 144:575–579.
Lloyd JR, Mirkov M. Selective photothermolysis of the sebaceous glands
    for acne treatment. Lasers Surg Med 2002; 31:115–120.
Mills OH, Kligman AM. Ultraviolet phototherapy and photochemotherapy
    of acne vulgaris. Arch Dermatol 1978; 114:221–223.
Orringer JS, Kang S, Hamilton T, Schumacher W, Cho S, Hammerberg C,
    Fisher GJ, Karimipour DJ, Johnson TM, Vorhees JJ. Treatment of
    acne vulgaris with a pulsed dye laser: a randomized controlled trial.
    J Am Med Assoc 2004; 291(23):2834–2839.
Paithankar DY, Ross EV, Saleh BA, Blair MA, Graham BS. Acne treat-
    ment with a 1,450 nm wavelength laser and cryogen spray cooling.
    Lasers Surg Med 2002; 31:106–114.
Papageorgiou P, Katsambas A, Chu A. Phototherapy with blue (415 nm)
    and red (660 nm) light in the treatment of acne vulgaris. Br J
    Dermatol 2000; 142:973–978.
Patton T, Kress D. Light therapy in the treatment of acne vulgaris. Cosmet
    Dermatol 2004; 17:373–378.
Tzung TY, Wu KH, Huang ML. Blue light therapy in the treatment of acne.
    Photodermatol Photoimmunol Photomed 2004; 20:266–269.

Practicing Photomedicine

There are several aspects of phototherapy and photochemotherapy that are quite different from other areas of dermatology practice, and providing these treatments is not just like adding another examination room. Decisions must be made about equipment that requires some knowledge about physics and engineering. Staff have to be trained to use the equipment. New fee schedules have to be developed and detailed records must be kept. These decisions and problems appear formidable at first glance but can be readily surmounted.

The first decision to be made is which type of facility you require: a day-care facility offering Goeckerman treatment or an ambulatory facility offering only UVB phototherapy and PUVA therapy. A day-care facility involves a considerable investment of space, time, and money, and I will assume that any person considering this venture will spend some time visiting an established clinic to learn how to develop and run a center. Thus, this part will mainly be directed at the physician who plans to provide UVB and PUVA therapy and possibly laser treatments.

Patients coming for treatment regard it as a nuisance since it takes a large bite of time out of their lives. This needs to be kept in focus when creating and planning a facility since the requirements of these patients are different from patients coming occasionally to see a physician. They want to get in, be treated, and get out quickly. This influences decisions such as locating a facility near major roads, provision of adequate and preferably free parking, offering flexible hours, and running this part of the office on schedule.

25

Creating a Facility

INTRODUCTION

Establishing a new facility has a few key components. First, a decision must be made about space requirements and location. Second, equipment must be selected. Third, the services of an electrician and probably also a plumber and builder will be required. The electrician is an important element because he will probably be the best source for service in the future and, it is hoped, will be interested in tinkering with equipment. Finally, you need patience because all will not happen as planned.

SPACE

A treatment facility is best located with direct access to the waiting area so that the operator can see patients when they arrive. Ideally, it should be separate and away from where the physician is seeing patients. Patients do not have to be seen by the physician each time they are treated, but if he or she is easily accessible, expect numerous corridor consultations and questions. Air-conditioning, power, and plumbing requirements must be considered. Most stand-up units require access to 220 V power. If the unit is to be air-conditioned, this will require a supply of water and access to a drain.

Treatment Space

The type of equipment to be used dictates the area required for treatment. Most stand-up units require an area of 6 ft × 4 ft since they are about 4 ft in diameter and space is required for opening the door and accessing the rear of the unit. In addition, a dressing area of 4 ft × 4 ft is required so that the combined space is about 40 ft². A hand and foot unit requires about 4 ft × 6 ft. A bed unit requires about 8 ft × 12 ft, including a dressing area. When an operator is in the same room or more than one unit is in a room, the treatment area must be curtained off with drapes suspended from the ceiling. A few simple points often overlooked: a speckled beige carpet or wooden floor is best for concealing or cleaning up a shower of psoriatic scales. In the changing area a chair, coat hooks, mirror, shelf, and waste bin will be appreciated by patients.

If laser, focal light treatments or photodynamic treatment is being provided, a separate room may be required as these treatments require constant presence of the operator.

Storage Space

A treatment facility requires many supplies such as gowns, pillow cases, paper, and spare bulbs, and some provision must be made for storage of these items close to the location of the facility.

Waiting Space

The additional flow of patients created by the facility must be considered, particularly since it can be assumed that many will not arrive at their scheduled treatment time. The minimum time slot for a treatment is usually 15 min, which means four patients each hour for each piece of equipment.

EQUIPMENT

Rapid expansion of interest in phototherapy and photochemotherapy on the part of both physicians and patients has led to the entry of numerous manufacturers into the market for equipment. The result is a bewildering array of products. Confusion is made even worse by the fact that the manufacturers, not surprisingly, stress the distinctive features of their products, often with particular emphasis on gadgets, and tend to ignore the similarities among the various products that are available. However, this situation can be clarified to some extent by concentrating on the common features of the treatment systems and adjunctive equipment. A physician's requirements for radiation equipment will depend on many factors, such as the size of the patient population, the desire to use phototherapy and photochemotherapy, and, not least of all, the cost of the equipment.

The following brief discussion is aimed at providing information on the advantages and disadvantages of the available equipment so that a better-informed decision can be made as to what is best for a given clinic or practice.

Fluorescent bulbs

These are the essential components of most treatment systems because they are fairly cheap to install and run, and they are reliable, requiring minimal servicing.

Types

A variety of brand names are attached to bulbs, but all fluorescent treatment systems made in the United States are fitted with lamps containing phosphors that provide one of three types of emission spectra.

Narrowband UVB bulbs: These lamps have a very narrow emission spectrum centered at 311 nm (Fig. 1). They are made by Philips Lighting (USA, Somerset, NJ) and have the designation TL 100 W 01.

Broadband UVB bulbs: These lamps have not only a predominant emission in the UVB region, but also some shorter wavelengths in the UVC waveband and some longer UVA and visible light (Fig. 2). They are often termed sunlamp bulbs, are made by several firms, and carry the designation TL/12.

UVA bulbs: These lamps have a predominant emission in the 320–400 nm range and also emit a small amount of UVB and some visible light (Fig. 3). Several firms produce UVA lamps that are marketed for use with psoralens and they usually carry the designation of PUVA bulbs. There are many other types of UVA lamps available for use in industry and tanning salons and the emission spectra of such lamps will vary with the use. Thus, the name "UVA lamp" or "BL lamp" does not necessarily mean it is suitable for therapy; it must be labeled as a PUVA lamp or as being suitable for use in PUVA therapy.

Length

Bulbs are available in various lengths. Bulbs of 2 and 4 ft length are used in units designed for treating localized disease. Six-feet bulbs are used in whole-body irradiators. When measurements of the irradiance are made close to the bulb, it is found to decrease from the center toward the ends, so that the irradiance over the terminal 6–12 in. may be 20% less than at the center. The effect is relatively independent of the length of the bulbs, and therefore a small irradiator lined with 2 ft bulbs will provide a lower irradiance than a large irradiator lined with 6 ft bulbs of the same type unless the shorter bulbs are driven to provide a higher output.

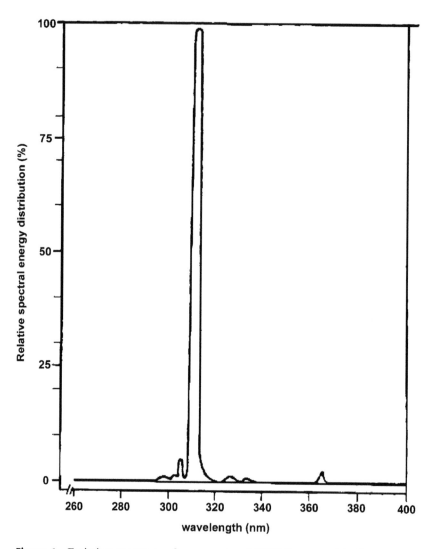

Figure 1   Emission spectrum of a narrowband UVB fluorescent bulb.

Life span

Various definitions can be used to describe the life span of fluorescent bulbs. The total life span until the bulb stops functioning is usually 3000 hr or more, a figure often used by manufacturers. However, the useful life span is much less and seldom exceeds 2000 hr. During the first few hours of use, the irradiance from a bulb declines rapidly, so that at 12 hr, the output has declined by 10–15%. The rate of decrease of the irradiance becomes less as the time increases (Fig. 4). The irradiance continues to decline fairly

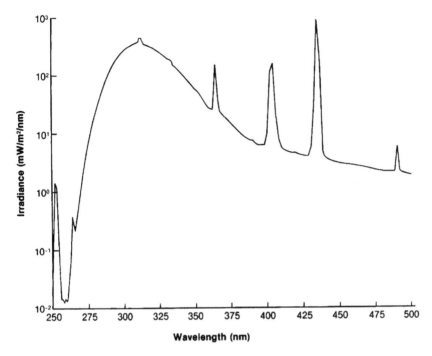

Figure 2 Emission spectrum of a broadband UVB fluorescent bulb.

rapidly for the first 100 hr, but at several hundred hours the decline is slow. Although the specific time course depends on the type of lamp and its ballasting, many lamps used in therapy can drop to <50% of their initial output by 2000 hr. The decision as to when to relamp will largely depend on the nature of the clinic and the patient load. Two approaches are commonly used: changing lamps when they cease to function or total relamping at a set age of 1000 or 2000 hr.

Run-in Time

A practical implication of the rapid decline in the output of bulbs in the first few hours of operation is that it is difficult to treat patients safely during that time without very frequent monitoring of the irradiance. One solution to this problem is to burn the bulbs for 12–24 hr, for example, by leaving the system on overnight, before using the system for treatment. Another solution is to use automatic radiometry, which will be discussed later in this chapter.

Warm-up Time

The output of bulbs also fluctuates during the first few minutes of operation due to increase in the temperature of the bulbs. However, except when

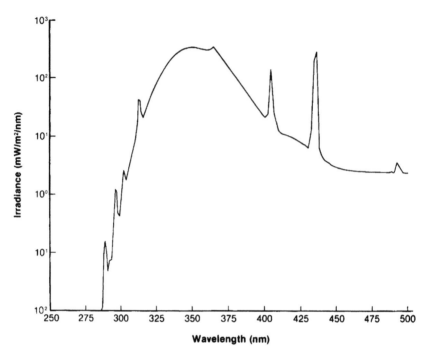

Figure 3   Emission spectrum of a PUVA fluorescent bulb.

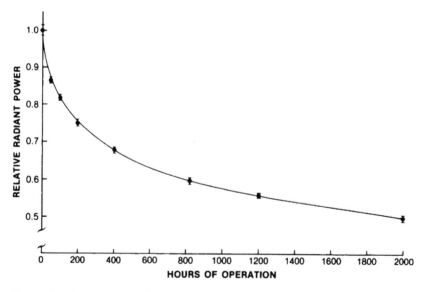

Figure 4   Time course of decline in irradiance of a PUVA fluorescent bulb.

taking measurements of the irradiance, this variation is unimportant and it is not necessary to "warm up" a radiator.

Ballasts

A ballast is an auxiliary electrical device that starts and provides proper electrical operation of a fluorescent lamp so that the output remains steady. Thus, the ballast is a major determinant of the irradiance of the lamp and in recent years electronic ballasts have been used that drive lamps above their rated operation to provide higher radiant power and therefore provide higher irradiance. This increase may or may not decrease the life span of the bulbs, depending on the details of the technique.

When a fluorescent lamp ceases to function it may be because the lamp has died or its ballast is defective. This is easy to distinguish: shift the lamp to an adjacent functioning socket and if it lights, the problem is the ballast.

Cost

Fluorescent lamps used in phototherapy probably cost less than $1 to make. UVA lamps cost less than $20. UVB lamps cost around $100. Why? I have not been able to find out, maybe it is a monopoly.

Metal Halide Lamps

Radiators are available that are equipped with metal halide lamps. These lamps provide a continuous emission spectrum from 280 nm through to visible radiation, as shown in Figure 5. However, two filters are provided to

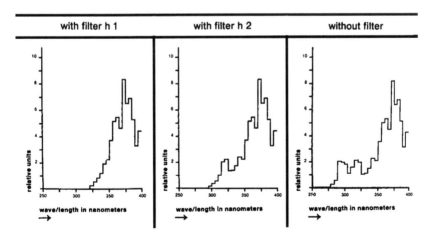

Figure 5 Emission spectrum of a metal halide lamp to provide UVA radiation (filter H1) (left), UVA and UVB radiation (filter H2) (middle), or the full spectrum of the lamp (without filter) (right).

restrict the emission spectrum to wavelengths >295 nm (UVB + UVA; Fig. 5, middle) or >315 nm (UVA; Fig. 5, left). The main advantage of these lamps is a high irradiance, which is at least double that of any fluorescent UVA or UVB bulb. Thus, treatment times are considerably shorter. The main disadvantage is cost, which is somewhat higher than that for fluorescent bulbs.

Radiators

Several types of radiators are available, and each has advantages and disadvantages depending on the requirements for therapy. A list of manufacturers of radiators is given in Table 1.

Table 1 Manufacturers of UV radiation systems

Cooper-Hewitt Corp., 20 Kenton Lands Road, Erlanger, KY 41018 (877) 289–2656, web address: www.homephototherapy.com
High-pressure mercury vapor lamp on a stand, suitable for local area treatment in the home or office
Daavlin, P.O. Box 626, Bryan, OH 43506, (800) 322–8546, web address: www.daavlin.com
Fluorescent stand-up units (UVA, UVB, UVA/UVB), hand and foot units, area units suitable for home or office
Environmental Growth Chambers, 510 East Washington Street, Chagrin Falls, OH 44022, (800) 321–6854, web address: www.egc.com
Fluorescent stand-up units (UVA, UVB)
National Biological Corporation, 1532 Enterprise Parkway, Twinsburg, OH 44087, (800) 338–5045), web address: www.natbiocorp.com
Fluorescent stand-up units (UVA, UVB, UVA/UVB), hand and foot units, area units suitable for home or office
Psoralite-Sunmaker, Inc., 2806 Wm. Tuller Drive, Columbia, SC 29205, (800) 331-3534
Fluorescent stand-up units (UVA, UVB, UVA/UVB) and area units suitable for home or office
Richmond Light Co., 2301 Falkirk Drive, Richmond, VA 23236, (888) 276–0559, web address: www.trlc.com, e-mail: trlc@trlc.com
Fluorescent UVB panels suitable for home use
Ultra-Derm Systems, 2201 South Michigan Avenue, Saginaw, MI 48602, (989) 792-6100
Fluorescent stand-up UVB units suitable for home or office
Ultraviolet Enterprises, 390 Farmer Court, Lawrenceville, GA 30245, (800) 241-7506, web address: www.ultralite-uv.com
Fluorescent stand-up units (UVA, UVB, UVA/UVB) with optional air-conditioning, a lie-down unit, a hand and foot unit with upper and lower panels, and area units suitable for home or office

---

Whole-Body Fluorescent Stand-Up Units

This is the most common type of radiator and suitable for most ambulatory patients. Units are fitted with varying numbers of bulbs, and the output increases with the increase in the number of bulbs. However, the relationship is not directly proportional, so that doubling the number of bulbs will increase the irradiance by something less than a factor of 2.

Types of bulbs: Units may be fitted with just one type of bulb or a combination of two types of bulbs. Commonly used configurations are

- Narrowband UVB unit containing 48 bulbs, which is optimal for this treatment since this will keep exposure times short.
- PUVA unit containing 48 UVA bulbs.
- A combination narrowband UVB/PUVA unit with 24 bulbs of each type. This is a useful compromise but treatment times will be longer.
- A combination PUVA/broadband UVB unit containing 40 UVA bulbs and 8 UVB bulbs. This is a useful unit since it will provide adequate output of both wavebands.

Uniformity of irradiance: If a unit is fitted with a full array of closely fitted bulbs around all sides, as is usual in UVA and narrowband radiators, there will be reasonable uniformity of irradiance with distance, or, put another way, all exposed surfaces will receive much the same dose in any horizontal plane. In such a unit the patient may stand still. In a combination unit some uniformity is sacrificed and patients should rotate during treatment.

Reflectors: An anodized aluminum reflector is usually located behind the bulbs to direct radiation back into the unit. This is an essential feature since it augments the irradiance by 20–40%.

Lamp containment: The patient must be protected from laceration if a bulb breaks during operation. The usual cause of breakage is the patient having a vaso-vagal syncope and falling against the lamps. Teflon sleeves, which transmit about 90% of the UV radiation, are available and these provide the best protection. In some units wire mesh is used to separate the patient from contact with bulbs, and this does prevent the patient from falling against the bulbs. However, this is not adequate, because it does not stop glass from falling on the floor if a lamp implodes.

Exposure control: Most units are equipped with a microprocessor or minicomputer to enter the treatment dose or time plus provide a variety of other functions. Simplicity and ease of operation are the main requirements. In some units the computer is used to store details about treatments and other patient data. In addition, it may be linked to a printer to provide a record for the patient's chart. This can result in the generation of a lot of paper.

Safety features: Hand-holds, patient-viewing windows or mirrors, nonslip floors, a switch to enable patients to stop a treatment, and safety doors appear to be standard on all equipment available.

Access for cleaning: Dust and scale readily collect in units and an important consideration is ease of access to reflector panels and other surfaces.

Problems: There are a few problems with stand-up units. First, the heat load generated is considerable and this will be discussed along with air-conditioning. Second, claustrophobia is a problem with some patients but this is greatly alleviated when the unit is open at the top. Third, due to reduced output at the ends of the bulbs the feet in particular and the head and neck in tall patients receive a reduced dose. Using a platform for the patient to stand on alleviates the problem for the feet but it exacerbates the problem for the head and neck in tall patients. Provision of a reflective panel above the unit might help to reduce this problem.

Metal Halide Stand-Up Units

There are some significant differences between these units and fluorescent systems, so they are worth separate consideration. Three columns, each containing five lamps, are contained in an enclosed unit with one control panel. This system appears to have two advantages. First, due to the reflector system behind the lamps the vertical irradiance is very uniform and does not fall at the top and bottom of the unit to any significant extent. Second, intrinsic to the lamp the output is high and treatment times are correspondingly shortened.

However, to balance these advantages there are a couple of disadvantages. Due to separation of the columns by a distance of 20 in, horizontal irradiance is very nonuniform. For UVA radiation, the irradiance in front of a column may be almost 70 mW/cm^2, but this falls to about 25 mW/cm^2 between the lamps. Thus, the patient must turn during the treatment and the shorter treatment time is partially translated into a lower actual dose. A second small problem is that the filters on the bulbs must be changed manually to switch from UVA to UVB treatment. If the correct filters are not in place, the wrong treatment will be given with risk of an erythema.

Lie-Down Fluorescent Units

These units have been widely used in Europe for therapy but have not been used much in the United States. However, they can be ordered here and therefore the advantages and disadvantages are worth consideration. A lie-down unit is obviously very useful for treating disabled patients who are unable to stand for the duration of a treatment. In addition, this unit is the only effective means of treating intertriginous areas and usually produces rapid clearance of disease in the groin and axillae. However, if the unit only has bulbs above the patient, treatment times are of course doubled. Finally, space is always important and a lie-down unit takes more floor space than a stand-up unit. Therefore, a lie-down unit is of interest mainly in a busy clinic with a sufficient number of patients who will benefit from its particular advantages.

Hand and Foot Units

These are extremely useful for adjunctive treatment of the palms and soles in patients also being treated in a stand-up unit, or for treatment of patients with disease confined to the hands and feet. Most units available appear to have overcome the early problem of a low output due to short fluorescent bulbs and the irradiance from these units is comparable to that of a stand-up unit. Two types of units are available. One type has bulbs in both the top and the bottom of each part of the hand and foot unit so that palms, soles, and the dorsa of the hands and feet can all be simultaneously treated. Other units only have bulbs in the bottom of each unit so that the dorsa of the feet cannot be treated and the palms and the dorsa of the hands must be treated separately.

It has already been noted that only PUVA therapy is effective in treating disease on the palms and soles in most cases. However, several manufacturers offer hand and foot units equipped with broadband and narrowband fluorescent UVB bulbs and I have had many physicians say "it must be effective because the equipment is available." If it were effective as a treatment there would be studies reporting this, but there are none. Of course this is not the first, nor will it be the last time physicians are offered equipment that does not produce the desired effect.

Area Units

Radiators are available that consist of a bank of fluorescent bulbs or a single metal halide bulb and are suitable for doing an MED or MPD or for treating local areas of disease. They can also be used as a hand or foot unit in some instances. One specialized device consists of a comb with a UVA bulb included, supposedly for treating scalp psoriasis but any response from its use would probably be due to a placebo effect, since the output of the unit is too low to have any significant biological effect.

Air-Conditioning

All radiators generate heat, and as a rule-of-thumb each fluorescent lamp emits heat equivalent to the body heat generated by one person. Therefore, the treatment facility must be air-conditioned and normal room air-conditioning is usually adequate to handle heat generated by area units and hand and foot units.

Stand-up units represent a different problem since they generate about 10,000 BTU/hr, which must be dissipated in some way. Imagine being surrounded by as many as 48 people, all within 2 ft of you, and this will give you some idea of the heat stress placed on patients in an inadequately cooled unit. One approach to the problem is to increase the room air-conditioning by 10,000 BTU, which, when combined with a fan in the unit, will control the ambient temperature and keep the temperature in the radiator around 90°F. Of course, in addition to providing air-conditioning, it must also be used, and this means an ambient temperature of about 55°F and sweaters for the staff. A better approach is to increase the room air-conditioning and vent air from the unit to the exterior. The best approach is to air-condition the units themselves.

Air conditioners available for stand-up units consist of a modified heat pump using water to carry away excess heat. One of these air conditioners can adequately cool three or four stand-up units via overhead ducting. The decision to air-condition the stand-up units will immediately result in a grateful response from patients, but be warned, as soon as they have forgotten how hot it used to be, they will start complaining that it is too cold!

Radiometers

The Equipment

A radiometer is a device used for measuring the irradiance of a source of photons. The radiometers used in therapy are often called photometers and the two terms are used interchangeably. There are several different types of radiometers, but in phototherapy, vacuum photodiodes are most commonly used because they have the features of low cost and simplicity and are fairly rugged. A radiometer system consists of two main components: a probe or sensor, and a measuring device for determining how many photons impinge on the probe. The probe has a characteristic spectral sensitivity, and those used by phototherapists are designed to measure narrowband UVB, broadband UVB, or broadband UVA radiation emitted by the three types of fluorescent bulbs that are available. Probes are not interchangeable, and measurements of the irradiance of a radiation source must be made with a probe that contains the appropriate filter for that source. The measuring device provides a reading for the irradiance in milliwatts per square centimeter , and it can be used with any probe, so it is only necessary to have one radiometer.

Handling and Calibration

Radiometers are fairly delicate instruments and should be handled with care. The instrument and probe must be stored in a protective casing, such as a box lined with foam rubber. If the instrument is dropped, malfunction will usually result, and it is then necessary to return it to the manufacturer for repair and recalibration. Even with normal use, a radiometer should be recalibrated every year or so.

Ideally, for a given radiation source, the measurements of irradiance obtained by all properly calibrated radiometers would be very similar. However, in the real world, this is far from true. The National Bureau of Standards has standard radiation sources available for calibrating radiometers, but some manufacturers appear to calibrate their product without proper reference to these standards. For example, it is common for one radiometer to give an irradiance measurement of 10 mW/cm^2 for a given radiation source and another radiometer to read 15 mW/cm^2. Accurate, consistent, and frequent radiometry is essential for the safe operation of a phototherapy unit. If in doubt about the accuracy of a radiometric reading, it is useful to have access to a second radiometer to provide a comparison.

Suppliers

Several of the manufacturers of UV radiation systems market radiometers, and, in addition, International Light, Inc. [Dexter Industrial Green, Newburyport, MA 01950 (617/465–5923)] manufactures and markets hand-held radiometers suitable for use with UVA and UVB treatment systems.

Techniques for Measurements

There are two approaches to radiometry: intermittent radiometry using a portable radiometer and automatic radiometry using a radiometer and probes that are built into the radiator. One system is not exclusive of the other and indeed the ideal arrangement is to use automatic radiometry with a safe alarm system and to have available a portable system for periodic checks.

Intermittent radiometry: A portable radiometer and the appropriate probe are used to measure the irradiance of the bulbs. Measurements should be made daily when the bulbs are new, and weekly when a plateau is reached. The duration of a given treatment can be calculated for each treatment, but it is much more convenient to construct a table of doses and irradiances as illustrated for UVA radiation in Table 2.

The conditions for taking measurements should be standardized as much as possible, with particular attention to having the radiator functioning for 5–10 min and placing the probe a set distance from the bulbs. One approach suitable for a UVA radiator is for a technician to stand inside the unit and take an irradiance measurement while pointing the sensor at the center of each of the panels of bulbs; the readings are then averaged to give the irradiance. The irradiance value when measured by a person standing in the unit will be 10–15% less than the actual irradiance because

Table 2 Duration[a] of UVA Treatments (min/sec) for Doses (J) Calculated for Various Irradiances (mW)

Dose (J/cm²)	Irradiances (mW)							
	15	16	17	18	19	20	21	22
1.0	1.07	1.02	0.59	0.56	0.53	0.50	0.48	0.46
1.5	1.40	1.34	1.28	1.23	1.19	1.15	1.11	1.08
2.0	2.13	2.05	1.58	1.51	1.45	1.40	1.35	1.31
2.5	2.47	2.36	2.27	2.19	2.11	2.05	1.59	1.53
3.0	3.20	3.08	2.56	2.47	2.38	2.30	2.23	2.16
3.5	3.53	3.39	3.26	3.14	3.04	2.55	2.47	2.39
4.0	4.26	4.10	3.55	3.42	3.31	3.20	3.11	3.02
4.5	5.00	4.41	4.25	4.10	3.57	3.45	3.34	3.25
5.0	5.34	5.13	4.54	4.38	4.23	4.10	3.58	3.47
5.5	6.07	5.44	5.23	5.05	4.49	4.35	4.22	4.10
6.0	6.40	6.15	5.53	5.34	5.16	5.00	4.46	4.33
6.5	7.13	6.46	6.22	6.01	5.42	5.25	5.10	4.56
7.0	7.47	7.17	6.52	6.29	6.08	5.50	5.34	5.18
7.5	8.20	7.49	7.21	6.56	6.35	6.15	5.57	5.41
8.0	8.53	8.20	7.50	7.25	7.01	6.40	6.21	6.04
8.5	9.26	8.51	8.20	7.52	7.28	7.05	6.45	6.26
9.0	10.00	9.23	8.49	8.20	7.53	7.30	7.08	6.49
9.5	10.34	9.54	9.19	8.48	8.20	7.55	7.32	7.12
10.0	11.07	10.25	9.48	9.16	8.46	8.20	7.56	7.35
10.5	11.40	10.56	10.17	9.43	9.13	8.45	8.20	7.58
11.0	12.13	11.28	10.47	10.11	9.39	9.10	8.44	8.20
11.5	12.47	11.59	11.16	10.39	10.05	9.35	9.08	8.43
12.0	13.20	12.30	11.46	11.07	10.32	10.00	9.32	9.05
12.5	13.53	13.01	12.15	11.34	10.58	10.25	9.55	9.28
13.0	14.26	13.32	12.45	12.02	11.24	10.50	10.19	9.51

[a]Minutes/seconds.

a body absorbs some of the radiation and reduces scattered radiation. Some units are supplied with a metal bracket that holds the sensor in the center of the unit, while the measurement is being taken, and this approach provides readings that are higher than those actually experienced by the patients in the unit. Provided the same technique is always used, either approach is satisfactory. Care must be taken when irradiance measurements for UVB radiation are being made because of the risk of erythema; these readings should be made rapidly by a fully protected person.

Automatic radiometry: Some radiators have a built-in probe and radiometer or, in the case of a combination UVA/UVB unit, two probes, one for each waveband. These radiometers are hooked into the control panel and provide constant monitoring of the output of the unit, which greatly enhances the accuracy of dosimetry. The dose of radiation is punched into the minicomputer and the machine delivers the exact dose regardless of the state of the lamps.

Automatic dosimetry with built-in radiometry is obviously a very convenient and accurate means of delivering treatment but there are three important provisos:

- Regular cleaning of the probe is essential since dirt and scale will settle on the surface resulting in a falsely low irradiance and, therefore, an incorrectly high exposure dose for the patient.
- The machine must be equipped with a shut-off device and an audible alarm in the event of a sudden reduction in irradiance. This usually occurs when the patient places their hand over the probe effectively reducing the reading close to zero so that the machine will keep going for a long time.
- The bulbs monitored by the probe should be checked daily to ensure that they are functioning correctly. The probe usually only monitors a few bulbs and it is necessary to check if they are representative of the condition of the rest of the unit using a hand-held radiometer.

Eye Protection

During Treatment

Eye protection is essential during both PUVA and UVB treatments. Small goggles that are UV-opaque and fit close to the skin around the eyes provide adequate protection and are available from manufacturers of radiators and other suppliers (Table 3). Large wraparound glasses provide protection but leave hypopigmented rings around the eyes and this is unacceptable to patients.

Table 3 Manufacturers of UV Protection Eyewear

Cooper-Hewitt Corp., 20 Kenton Lands Road, Erlanger, KY 41018, (877) BUY-AMJO, web address: www.homephototherapy.com
"DPE-1," plastic goggles for protection during treatment
Dioptics, 51 Zaca Lane, San Luis Obispo, CA 93401, (805) 781-3300, web address: www.dioptics.com, e-mail: info@dioptics.com
"Solarshield" wraparound plastic sunglasses, clear and in various colors; suitable to use alone or over glasses
Lucas Products Corp., P.O. Box 6570, Toledo, OH 43612, (419) 476-5992, web address: www.lucasproducts.com
"Sunnies" eyeshields, plastic goggles for protection during treatment
Noir Medical Technologies, P.O. Box 159, South Lyon, MI 48178, (800) 521-9746, web address: www.noir-medical.com
"UV shield" wraparound plastic sunglasses, clear and in various colors; suitable to use alone or over glasses

---

Before and After PUVA Therapy

The best protection is provided by wraparound glasses that are UV-opaque and clear or colored depending on patient preference (Table 3). Fashion-conscious patients may prefer to buy more stylish glasses such as Ray-Ban and this is perfectly acceptable. Some patients will be very resistant to using wraparound styles and application of a UV-opaque coating to the patient's own lenses is a reasonable compromise to ensure compliance.

Testing Glasses

When a patient insists on using his own glasses for eye protection before and after PUVA therapy, it is essential to confirm that they are UV-opaque. This can be readily accomplished by placing the glasses over the UVA probe of the radiometer while it is pointed at a source of UVA radiation. The reading should be close to zero if the glasses are opaque.

Electrical Connections

Most whole-body radiators require 40–60 A and 240 V power and usually the electrical inspector will insist it be hard-wired with a breaker at the wall. Most other equipment uses 120 V wall receptacles. Equipment may not be certified by a nationally recognized testing laboratory, such as UL, but there is usually no problem obtaining certification locally if that is requested by the inspector.

Conclusions

Radiators are the most expensive items for a therapy unit, and most physicians feel somewhat inadequate to the task of correctly evaluating the various brands available. However, an understanding of the characteristics of the equipment as outlined above, always remembering that the similarities among different brands are much more important than the differences, and a healthy degree of skepticism when presented with extravagant claims by salespeople usually will ensure a correct choice. Price has not been discussed because that is an individual decision. Service will vary with location, and no manufacturer seems to have emerged as outstanding in this regard; the small number of companies involved probably precludes uniform nationwide service. However, the equipment is simple and reliability does not appear to be a major problem.

BIBLIOGRAPHY

Ultraviolet Lamps

Diffey BL. The spectral emissions from ultraviolet radiation lamps used in dermatology. Photodermatology 1986; 3:179–185.
Diffey BL, Farr PM. An appraisal of ultraviolet lamps used for the phototherapy of psoriasis. Br J Dermatol 1987; 117:49–56.
Fischer T, Alsins J, Berne B. Ultraviolet-action spectrum and evaluation of ultraviolet lamps for psoriasis healing. Int J Dermatol 1984; 23:633–637.
Morison WL, Pike RA. Spectral power distributions of radiation sources used in phototherapy and photochemotherapy. J Am Acad Dermatol 1984; 10:64–68.
Mutzhas MF, Holzle E, Hofmann C, Plewig G. A new apparatus with high radiation energy between 320–460 nm: physical description and dermatological applications. J Invest Dermatol 1981; 76:42–47.

Radiators

Androphy EJ, Eaglstein WH. UV-B—energy distribution of phototherapy equipment. Arch Dermatol 1984; 120:17–18.
Bickford ED. Risks associated with use of UV-A irradiators being used in treating psoriasis and other conditions. Photochem Photobiol 1979; 30:199–202.
Chue B, Borok M, Lowe NJ. Phototherapy units: comparison of fluorescent ultraviolet B and ultraviolet A units with a high-pressure mercury system. J Am Acad Dermatol 1988; 18:641–645.
Mountford PJ. Phototherapy and photochemotherapy ultraviolet irradiation equipment. Photodermatology 1986; 3:83–91.

Radiometry

Diffey BL, Harrington TR, Challoner AVJ. A comparison of the anatomical uniformity of irradiation in two different photochemotherapy units. Br J Dermatol 1978; 99:361.

Diffey BL, Roelandts R. Status of ultraviolet A dosimetry in methoxsalen plus ultraviolet A therapy. J Am Acad Dermatol 1986; 15:1209–1213.

Fanselow D, Crone M, Dahl MV. Dosimetry in phototherapy cabinets. J Am Acad Dermatol 1987; 17:74–77.

Protection

Davey JB, Diffey BL, Miller JA. Eye protection in psoralen photochemotherapy. Br J Dermatol 1981; 104:295–300.

Moseley H, Cox NH, Mackie RM. The suitability of sunglasses used by patients following ingestion of psoralen. Br J Dermatol 1988; 118:247–253.

Moseley H, Diffey BL, Marks JM, et al. Personal solar UV-A doses received by patients undergoing oral psoralen photochemotherapy for psoriasis. Br J Dermatol 1981; 105:573.

Morison WL, Strickland PT. Environmental UVA radiation and eye protection during PUVA therapy. J Am Acad Dermatol 1983; 9:522–525.

Wennersten G. Photoprotection of the eye in PUVA therapy. Br J Dermatol 1978; 98:137–139.

26

Operating a Facility

INTRODUCTION

The main goal in operating a facility that offers UV therapy is to provide safe and effective treatment. This can be achieved by a physician who understands the treatment, working with staff who know how to deliver the treatments, and using equipment that is safe and reliable. Perhaps it is a reflection on the state of medicine, but certainly we must add a second goal in operating a facility and that is to make it financially viable. The number of physicians offering phototherapy in the United States plunged during the 1990s as costs rose and reimbursement rates stagnated. Therefore, decisions about which treatment to offer and how to charge for them must be based on sound financial decisions.

PHYSICIAN TRAINING

In an ideal world all residents in dermatology would receive full training in all aspects of photomedicine with a great deal of supervised hands-on experience in therapy. For those residents who are not part of this ideal world and older physicians, symposia on therapy at the annual meeting of the American Academy of Dermatology offer a partial substitute. Membership in the Photomedicine Society, which meets the day before the annual meeting of the AADA, is another source of education about phototherapy and this comes with a subscription to *Photodermatology, Photoimmnology, and Photomedicine*, a useful journal for physicians interested in phototherapy.

STAFF

The staff members who actually dispense the treatment are a major factor in determining the response of patients to therapy. If it is assumed that anybody who happens to be around at the time can act as a phototherapy technician, mistakes will be made and results will be poor. There are certain considerations that apply regardless of whether treatment is being delivered in a large, busy clinic or an office with only a small patient load.

Selection

The ideal persons for delivering treatment are trained nurses because these people know how to communicate with and motivate patients; they place emphasis on attention to detail, which is essential for good therapy, and are trained to keep good records, another essential. There is a shortage of nurses across the country but positions in doctors' offices are popular away from the stresses of working in a busy hospital. I have found that employing parttime nurses who work one day a week is a very successful approach to staffing since then they cover for each other and this circumvents problems of sick leave and vacations. Of course, this makes communications between the staff of paramount importance. Due to cost considerations, many physicians will elect not to employ nurses, and in this case the other considerations to be outlined, such as training and motivation, become more important.

Training

The staff must be thoroughly educated about the disease being treated, the nature of the treatment, and the likely response to the treatment. Emphasis must be placed on the dangers of making errors and the need for calling the physician's attention to any unusual occurrences. A new staff member usually needs a week or more of training before being given full responsibility for treatment. The National Psoriasis Foundation conducts courses around the country several times each year for educating phototherapy nurses and technicians and these are a very valuable means of training staff.

Motivation

The staff must be strongly motivated toward helping people and interested in the numerous minor problems that patients present to them. Patients must not be made to feel that they are a product passing along an assembly line. Both the treatment staff and the front-office staff must remember they are dealing with patients who already have a chronic disease with all the disability that it causes and who are now being asked to engage in a very demanding treatment schedule. Even when patients are responding well to treatment, they tend to get burnout and need support and encouragement.

Communication

When more than one technician is involved in treating patients, efficient lines of communication must be established. A logbook recording events occurring during the day is part of such a system, but oral communication is also important. For example, the time when units are being relamped can be a dangerous period. All technicians must be told about the current status of each unit; otherwise, it is quite possible that patients will be overtreated because of an incorrect assumption that the irradiance of the units is unchanged. Such oral communication is routine in a hospital setting among nurses but may be quite new to an office practice.

SCHEDULING OF PATIENTS

A small office with only a few patients might operate on a walk-in basis, but in most instances it is necessary to have an appointment system. Use of 15 and 30 min timeslots is most convenient. Treatments of <10 min duration are booked for 15 min and longer treatments require 30 min to allow time for undressing and dressing. Constant features of the schedule are early and late arrivals, patients taking their psoralen at the wrong time, and "no-shows." Continual admonishment by the staff with support from the physician is essential to keep these problems at a tolerable level. Because of these problems, in a busy clinic with multiple units it is only possible to book for three of four units, the fourth unit providing a reserve to compensate for the erratic behavior of the patients. From a staffing viewpoint such an arrangement also works well because four whole-body units plus one or two hand and foot units is the maximum number that can be handled by one staff member.

In the age of computers, scheduling of phototherapy appointments is one instance where a computer is not effective. Many patients will make one, two, or even three changes to their treatment time during the course of a day and this is best handled by using a penciled log.

RECORDS

Good records of the history and treatment of patients are always essential, but there are some aspects of this task with UVB phototherapy and PUVA therapy that require special mention. There are several reasons for this emphasis.

- The treatments are dispensed by the physician, who is therefore the sole source of information about which treatment was given to a patient.
- The treatments involve medical devices, and the function of these must be recorded.

- PUVA therapy is frequently used in a manner somewhat contrary to the guidelines that have been published. Familiarity with these guidelines is essential, and careful records must be kept of the treatment of patients when the guidelines are breached.
- The long-term effects of some of these treatments are unknown, and therefore records could be useful for future evaluation of the therapy.

The types of records that should be kept are as follows.

Initial Evaluation

A standard form is useful for recording the history and examination of the patient, and this has been discussed under the evaluation of the patient. A checklist is also advisable so that there is a record that an eye examination was performed, blood tests were done, and the details of the treatment and precautions to be taken were explained to the patient. The exact content of the form and checklist can be tailored to the physician's needs. Opinions differ as to whether it is necessary to have patients sign a consent form. The most important considerations are that the treatment has been explained, including its adverse effects and potential benefit plus, ideally, a handout has been provided and the patient has been given an opportunity to ask questions. If all this is documented, a consent form is probably superfluous and certainly not a substitute for these actions.

Progress Evaluations

Circumstances will differ with the type of clinic or practice that is the setting for therapy, but some guidelines can be suggested for evaluation of the progress of patients. During the clearance phase of treatment, the patient should be seen by a physician after every 6–10 treatments or more frequently if the patient is having problems with the treatment. A record of these evaluations should be kept. During the maintenance phase, the need for frequent evaluations diminishes, but again an evaluation every 6–10 treatments is suitable or a minimum of every 3–4 months in patients on monthly treatments. In busy clinics, care must be taken that patients do not become lost in the system and, as a result, direct their own treatment. If the patient is responding well, this can be a very real temptation, but the end result is usually excessive exposure to therapy. Before each treatment, all patients should be seen by an informed technician or nurse and a note made of their progress; these comments are most conveniently made on the treatment flowsheets.

Treatment Record

Sample flowsheets for UVB, PUVA therapy, and combination UVB/PUVA therapy are illustrated in Figures 1–3. In many ways, these are the most

UVB TREATMENT SHEET

Name:_____

Telephone # Home:_____   Telephone # Office: _____

Diagnosis: _____   Protocol: _____

SkinType: _____   MED: _____

Date	Day	Rx #	TRUNK		ARMS AND LEGS		SHIELD		Clin Appt	Comments
			J/cm^2 Total J/cm^2	Time Min	J/cm^2 Total J/cm^2	Time Min	Face	Other		

Figure 1 Flowsheet for UVB phototherapy.

crucial portions of the record on the patient, as they are usually the key to solving problems with therapy. The flowsheet is a record of what probably happened and much more reliable than the recollection of a patient. Patients will frequently overstate their reliability in attending for treatments, while the flowsheet will provide an accurate record of attendance. To augment the value of the record, a good practice is to enter all scheduled treatments, and then if the patient does not attend due to cancellation or is a no-show, the treatment is lined through and a notation of C for cancellation or NS for no-show is added (Fig. 4). Problems are quickly detected in this way. Physician's orders should be entered on the flowsheet and highlighted for ease of reading. Finally, each time the patient is evaluated by the physician should be noted on the flowsheet so that patients who are avoiding the

PUVA TREATMENT SHEET

Name: _____

Telephone # Home: _____   Telephone # Office: _____

Diagnosis: _____   Protocol: _____

Skin Type: _____   MPD: _____   Methoxsalen Dose: _____

| Date | Rx # | TRUNK | | ARMS AND LEGS | | SHIELD | | Clin Appt | Comments |
		J/cm^2 Total J/cm^2	Time Min	J/cm^2 Total J/cm^2	Time Min	Face	Other		

Figure 2 Flowsheet for PUVA therapy.

physician can be detected before they go too long conducting their own treatment.

Treatment System

The history of the treatment system should be recorded. Important points to be noted are as follows:

1. Date of the first operation.
2. Date of relamping and the number of hours of operation of the lamps.

PUVA TREATMENT SHEET

Name: _____

Diagnosis: _____ **Protocol:** _____

Skin Type: _____ **Methoxsalen Dose:** _____

Date	Rx #	TRUNK		ARMS AND LEGS		SHIELD		Clin Appt	Comments
		J/cm^2 / Total J/cm^2	Time Min	J/cm^2 / Total J/cm^2	Time Min	Face	Other		

UVB TREATMENT SHEET

Date	Rx #	TRUNK		ARMS AND LEGS		SHIELD		Clin Appt	Comments
		J/cm^2 / Total J/cm^2	Time Min	J/cm^2 / Total J/cm^2	Time Min	Face	Other		

Figure 3 Flowsheet for combination PUVA/UVB therapy.

3. Date of any major alterations to the radiator.
4. Date of calibration of radiometers.
5. If intermittent radiometry is being used, the irradiance of the system should be recorded at least weekly and more often with new bulbs.

SUPPLIES

There are a few items that are somewhat unique to UV therapy.

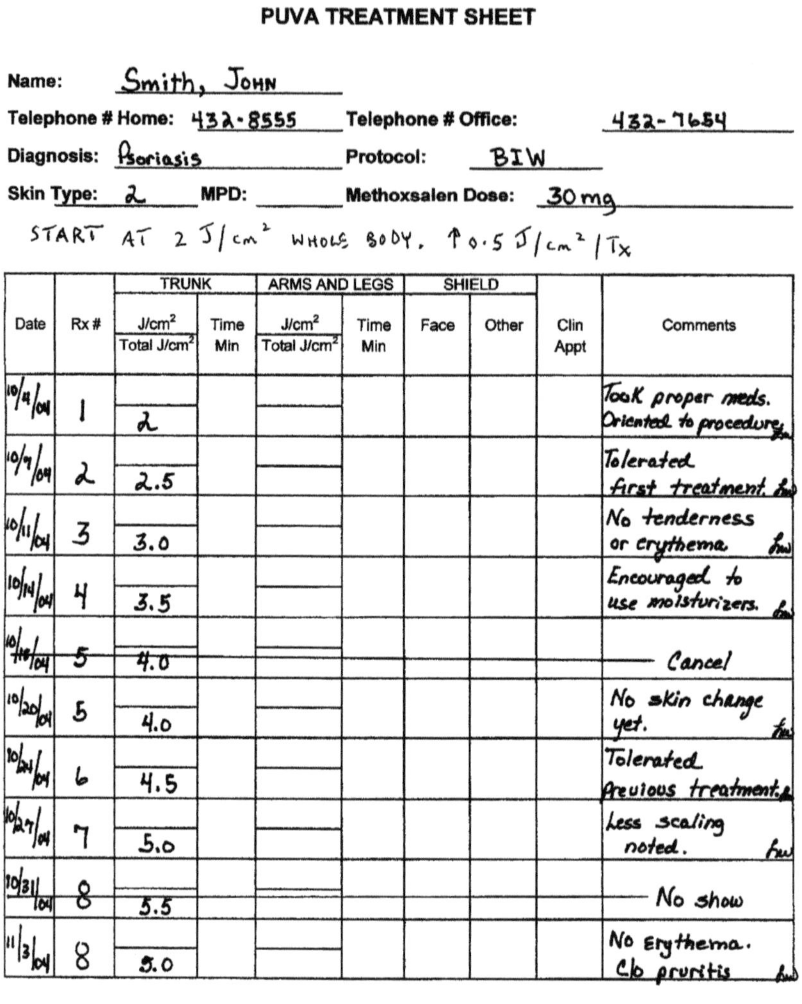

PUVA TREATMENT SHEET

Name: Smith, John

Telephone # Home: 432-8555   **Telephone # Office:** 432-7654

Diagnosis: Psoriasis   **Protocol:** BIW

Skin Type: 2   **MPD:** _____   **Methoxsalen Dose:** 30 mg

START AT 2 J/cm² WHOLE BODY. ↑ 0.5 J/cm²/Tx

Date	Rx #	TRUNK J/cm² / Total J/cm²	Time Min	ARMS AND LEGS J/cm² / Total J/cm²	Time Min	SHIELD Face	Other	Clin Appt	Comments
10/9/04	1	2							Took proper meds. Oriented to procedure.
10/9/04	2	2.5							Tolerated first treatment.
10/11/04	3	3.0							No tenderness or erythema
10/14/04	4	3.5							Encouraged to use moisturizers.
10/16/04	5	4.0							———— Cancel
10/20/04	5	4.0							No skin change yet.
10/24/04	6	4.5							Tolerated previous treatment.
10/27/04	7	5.0							Less scaling noted.
10/31/04	8	5.5							———— No show
11/3/04	8	5.0							No Erythema. C/o pruritis

Figure 4   Example of use of flowsheet.

Gowns and Pillowcases

These are required for giving extra treatment to the limbs. Blue snowflake gowns that overlap and tie are the most suitable gowns. Gowns with clips gape along the line of closure and disposable gowns do not fold and roll up satisfactorily. Pillowcases are required for protection of the head; the local discount store is usually the best source for these as their price is half that of hotel supply houses.

Disposable Underpads

These are required for providing a clean surface for the patient to stand on for whole-body treatment. The 24 in × 24 in size fits most units.

Sunscreens

Sunscreens are necessary for application to the face during treatment, and various manufacturers are willing to provide samples for this purpose. A supply of zinc oxide ointment is also necessary for application to areas of local erythema.

Moisturizers

Moisturizers are essential for UVB treatments and probably also for PUVA treatments, although this has not been established in clinical trials. Some patients may prefer to bring their own.

Nail Polish and Remover

These are necessary for patients who develop photo-onycholsis.

Cleaning Supplies

The treatment units should be cleaned daily using a germicidal cleanser such as Super Sani-cloth® disposable wipes.

NEWSLETTER

Many physicians now use a newsletter as a means of building goodwill and for marketing their practice. In a photomedicine office or clinic it can perform several other functions because the number of patients is fairly small, they only have a few diseases, and the treatments are fairly uniform. Useful functions for a newsletter include the following:

- Warnings about potential problems or adverse effects. For example, patients can be informed about the problem of spontaneous rupture of Oxsoralen Ultra capsules or the report of a high incidence of genital skin cancer in males, with advice about precautions that should be taken.
- Information about recent developments in research and treatment of psoriasis and other diseases being treated.
- Requests that patients keep their appointments, call to cancel when not coming, and are on schedule.
- News about changes in staff, office hours, or the treatment being provided.

In this way a newsletter can be a very effective means of increasing the safety and efficacy of the treatment.

SUPPORT GROUPS

In a large facility there is the opportunity to organize support groups among interested patients. These can be organized by the nurse conducting the treatment with occasional attendance by the physician. In addition, making patients aware of national organizations interested in their particular disease can be therapeutic in itself. The groups of interest are listed in Table 1.

ECONOMIC CONSIDERATIONS

The establishment of a unit providing phototherapy and photochemotherapy requires an expenditure of money, time, and effort on the part of the physician. Therefore, it is necessary to consider carefully the benefits that might be derived from such a unit, the potential demand for its services, the types of unit that will be most suitable, and the likely costs involved.

Benefits of Providing Therapy

The physician may benefit in several ways by providing PUVA and UVB phototherapy within a clinic or office practice. First, if these services are available nearby, it is likely that patients will be lost from the practice if they are not provided. Second, the provisions of these services will broaden the interest of the practice, as does any new innovation in medicine. Third, the service is likely to generate additional income, provided there is sufficient demand for it and the composition of the unit has been correctly matched to that demand. These benefits are self-evident but are stated so that the relative importance of each in making a decision to provide phototherapy or photochemotherapy within a practice will be given due consideration. The first two benefits may be obtained regardless of whether the service returns a profit, while the third benefit requires careful consideration of the remaining points raised in this section.

Demand for Therapy

The demand for PUVA and UVB therapy will depend on the number of diseases that are being treated and the size of the available population of patients with those diseases. Obviously, if these treatments are not available in the immediate vicinity, a population of referred patients may also be considered. There are several variables that influence the demand for UV radiation therapy.

Table 1 Associations Interested in Various Diseases

Eczema Association for Science and Education, 4460 Redwood Hwy, Ste. 16-D, San Rafael, CA 94903-1953, e-mail: info@nationaleczema.org, web address: www.nationaleczema.org

Mycosis Fungoides Foundation, P.O. Box 374, Birmingham, MI 48012-0374, e-mail: info@mffoundation.org, web address: www.mffoundation.org

National Psoriasis Foundation, 6600 SW 92nd Ave., Suite 300, Portland OR 97223-7195, e-mail: getinfo@psoriasis.org, web address: www.psoriasis.org

National Vitiligo Foundation, 700 Olympic Plaza Circle, Suite 404, Tyler, TX 75701, e-mail: vitiligo@vitiligofoundation.org, web address: www.nvfi.org

Patient Characteristics

An intelligent and settled patient population is ideal for these treatments. Conversely, poorly educated or transient patients are usually unsuitable and likely to have very great fluctuations in their demand for this service.

Insurance Coverage

The ability of patients to pay for treatment must be considered in all but the most wealthy of patient populations; this will be largely determined by insurance coverage. In most areas, Medicare, Medicaid, and private insurance carriers pay for phototherapy and PUVA therapy when used for ambulatory patients. However, HMOs provide variable coverage and some refuse to provide these treatments. The disease being treated is an important factor in determining insurance coverage. Most carriers reimburse for psoriasis, eczema, and vitiligo without question. Coverage for other diseases may be denied but this is often reversed when the physician sends a letter to the carrier explaining the medical necessity for the treatment. It is important to include in this letter a discussion of alternative treatments, if any are available, why UV therapy is the best choice and to attach a reprint of at least one reference to a study supporting use of the treatment.

Seasonal Variation

There is marked seasonal variation in demand for treatment in patients with psoriasis. Peak demand is in spring since patients want to be clear for the summer and then demand declines considerably during the summer months because most patients with psoriasis respond to sunlight as a therapy. This effect is most marked in colder climates while in warm climates overall demand is likely to be lower but more constant throughout the year.

Operating Hours

The hours when treatment is available has a significant impact on demand because most patients have to fit treatments into their work, school, or social schedule. Early morning, lunchtime, and early evening are the most popular times during the week and weekend hours can also be popular. If the service is only available from 9 a.m. to 5 p.m. 5 days a week, demand will be much less than if more flexible hours of operation are provided.

Alternate Treatments

Present and future alternate treatments must be considered, since they will influence demand for these services. However, the effect of a new treatment on demand may be difficult to predict. For example, the publicity associated with introduction of biologic drugs for treatment of psoriasis appears to have increased demand for UV therapy by causing patients who had given up on treatment to visit and find out about the new agents and instead many of them decide to try a course of UV therapy.

Type of Therapy

The demand for treatment in most small office practices will only support a single stand-up unit and the best choice in these circumstances is a combination unit containing either 24 narrowband UVB and 24 UVA bulbs or 8 broadband UVB and 40 UVA bulbs. Disease on the palms and soles can be treated by seating the patient in front of one UVA panel. A larger office might support one 48-bulb narrowband UVB unit, one combination unit with 40 UVA bulbs and 8 broadband UVB bulbs, and a hand/foot area unit.

Costs

The cost of providing UV therapy is largely fixed and does not fluctuate greatly with demand. The costs involved in establishing and maintaining a small facility equipped with one radiator are outlined in Table 2. This facility could provide 50 treatments per week, but it is assumed that only 20 treatments are given weekly. At that level of use, a net collection of about $29 per treatment would be required to cover costs. The costs of a larger facility are outlined in Table 3. This facility could provide 100 or more treatments each week but a more realistic level of activity of 60 treatments

Table 2 Cost of Phototherapy Facility with One Radiator

	Cost/year ($)
Radiator and renovations	
Radiator	2,142
Renovations	2,400
Maintenance and relamping	2,786
Interest	4,320
Personnel	
20% of technician	5,000
5% of physician	7,500
Space	
100 ft^2 at $25/ft^2	2,500
Billing and record keeping	
$3/visit	3,120
Total costs	29,766

Note: Cost are based on a facility equipped with one radiator, using part-time staff, and assuming straight-line depreciation over 7 years. Physician time applies only to administration and excludes times involved caring for patients directly.

Table 3 Cost of Phototherapy Facility with Two Stand-Up Radiators and a Hand/Foot Unit

	Cost/year ($)
Radiator and renovations	
Radiator	4,857
Renovations	4,800
Maintenance and relamping	6,208
Interest	7,440
Personnel	
One to two full-time technicians	30,000
10% of physicians	15,000
Space	
250 ft^2 at $25/ft^2	6,250
Billing and recordkeeping	
$3/visit	9,360
Total costs	83,915

Note: Costs are based on a facility equipped with two radiators, using full-time staff, and assuming straight-line depreciation over 7 years. Physician time for administration only.

per week has been used for the calculations. A net collection of $27 per treatment would be required to cover costs. The actual costs will vary with circumstances and miscellaneous costs for supplies, electricity, telephones, and the like have not been included in the calculations.

It is important for a physician to have a clear idea of his or her actual cost for delivery of UV therapies since this will be important when negotiating contracts with third-party payers. It is quite common for an insurance carrier to offer good reimbursement for most dermatology codes while reimbursing at a level well below cost for UV therapies. Some physicians counter that the marginal cost of providing more treatments is much less than the average cost of treatment and that is true as long as the marginal cost is not suddenly escalated by having to add more staff and equipment.

Coding

There are four CPT codes for phototherapy and photochemotherapy and these are listed in Table 4. Code 96900 is an old code and is seldom used today. Since both broadband and narrowband UVB phototherapies are clearly enhanced by prior application of petrolatum or other moisturizer, the correct code for these treatments is 96910. Code 96912 for PUVA therapy is self-explanatory. Code 96913 is used by psoriasis day-care centers. In addition to the code used for the treatment some centers also code a bill for the pretreatment evaluation by the nurse using code 99211 and modifier.

Table 4 CPT Codes (2004) for Phototherapy and Photochemotherapy

96900	Actinotherapy (UV light)
96910	Photochemotherapy, tar, and UVB (Goeckerman treatment) or petrolatum and UVB
96912	Psoralens and UVA (PUVA)
96913	Photochemotherapy (Goeckerman and/or PUVA) for severe photoresponsive dermatoses requiring at least four to eight hours of care under direct supervision of the physician (includes application of medication and dressings)

The cost of physician time and input to treatment can be recovered in various ways. Reimbursement by Medicare for the phototherapy and photo-chemotherapy codes does not include a physician component. Therefore, follow-up visits by the physician should be coded using evaluation and management codes and for an uncomplicated follow-up visit code 99212 appears appropriate; when the patient is treated on the same day this will require modifier 25. Most insurance carriers have switched to this approach and are following the lead provided by Medicare. However, some carriers are still only reimbursing for a bundled charge that includes physician time and effort in the single charge for the treatment.

REGULATIONS

Fortunately, there are few regulations that specifically impact on the physician providing UV therapy but a couple should be noted.

FDA Approval

There is sometimes confusion about the approved uses for PUVA therapy and this is mainly due to changes in products. The indications approved by the FDA are

- Oxsoralen Ultra capsules for psoriasis
- 8-MOP capsules for psoriasis and vitiligo
- Oxsoralen lotion for vitiligo.

Oral PUVA therapy is approved for treatment in an office or clinic under the direct supervision of a physician and it is not approved for home use. When using Oxsoralen lotion the drug should be applied by the physician.

Medicare Reimbursement

Medicare (Center for Medicare and Medicaid services) regulations require the physician responsible for the care of the patient to be in the immediate vicinity when treatment is being given, in order to qualify for reimbursement. This stipulation does not appear to apply to private insurance carriers.

Index